Dr. Abdulaziz Abdulshakoor Howsawi is a Family Medicine Physician who currently lives in Saudi Arabia, Riyadh. Abdulaziz likes to spend his free time reading, exercising, and watching movies. His inspiration to write this book comes from his residency program that he attends in Family Medicine. Goals and dreams for himself include living a healthy lifestyle and writing a personal development book.

To my Parents:
I could never have done this without your prayers, support, and constant encouragement.
Dad! I hope you are happy up there in heaven.

To my Wife and Children:
You are my life … my heart … my happiness … my world … my everything.

To my Siblings:
My world is full of smiles, whenever you are with me.

Dr. Abdulaziz Abdulshakoor Howsawi

SUMMARY OF COMMON CONDITIONS IN FAMILY MEDICINE

AUSTIN MACAULEY PUBLISHERS™
LONDON * CAMBRIDGE * NEW YORK * SHARJAH

Copyright © Dr. Abdulaziz Abdulshakoor Howsawi 2024

The right of Dr. Abdulaziz Abdulshakoor Howsawi to be identified as author of this work has been asserted by the author in accordance with Federal Law No. (7) of UAE, Year 2002, Concerning Copyrights and Neighboring Rights.

All rights reserved. No part of this publication may be reproduced, stored in a retrieval system, or transmitted in any form or by any means, electronic, mechanical, photocopying, recording, or otherwise, without the prior permission of the publishers.

Any person who commits any unauthorized act in relation to this publication may be liable to legal prosecution and civil claims for damages.

The medical information in this book is not advice and should not be treated as such. Do not substitute this information for the medical advice of physicians. The information is general and intended to better inform readers of their health care. Always consult your doctor for your individual needs.

The age group that matches the content of the books has been classified according to the age classification system issued by the Ministry of Culture and Youth.

ISBN - 9789948779889 - (Paperback)
ISBN - 9789948779896 - (E-Book)

Application Number: MC-10-01-1245977
Age Classification: E

First Published 2024
AUSTIN MACAULEY PUBLISHERS FZE
Sharjah Publishing City
P.O Box [519201]
Sharjah, UAE
www.austinmacauley.ae
+971 655 95 202

There are countless people I would like to thank for their help throughout my life, without whom I would not be able who I am or doing what I do. For the sake of brevity here, I would like to acknowledge and thank those who have had the greatest impact on the success of this book.

My deepest gratitude goes to Dr. Sulaiman AlAqeel, Dr. Moath AlKathiri, Dr. Abdulrahman AlYemni, Dr. Salman AlDakhil, and Dr. Omar AlSughayir, for being there always whenever I need them. Many thanks to Dr. Abdulrahman AlShebel, Dr. Nasser Muharib, Dr Hamzah AlKhalifah, Dr. Yazeed ElZahrany, and Dr. Homood AlShahrani for their support in writing this book. I am indebted to my colleagues in Family Medicine Residency Program, Dr. Abdulelah AlMutairi, Dr. Faisal AlDosari, Dr. Hamzah AlOtaibi, Dr. Naif AlRudhaian, Dr. Ali AlQahtani, Dr. Ahmad AlGhamdi, Dr. Abdullah AlOwayed, Dr. Esam Quqandi, Dr. Mohanned AlAhmari, Dr. Mutlaq AlMutlaq, Dr. Ammar AlMulhim, and Dr. Zaid AlShareef for their time and thoughts. I extend special thanks to Dr. Ahmad Selaihem, Dr. Mamdouh AlOtaibi, Dr. Mishary AlMishary, Dr. Khalid AlRashed, Dr. Akram AlHazmi, Dr. Saleh AlHazmi, Dr. Bandar AlShehry and Dr. Noorul Zaman Kadher for their efforts during my residency program in Family Medicine.

Table of Contents

Section 1: Cardiovascular — 15
    Heart Failure — 17
    Hypertension — 24
    Dyslipidemia — 27
    Acute Coronary Syndrome — 28
    Palpitation — 33
    Atrial Fibrillation — 37
    Giant Cell Arteritis — 40
    Chads$_2$ Score — 42
    Has-Bled Score — 43
    NOAC Anticoagulation — 44
    Pulseless Electrical Activity (PEA) — 45

Section 2: Dermatology — 47
    Acne Vulgaris — 49
    Atopic Dermatitis — 53
    Contact Dermatitis — 55
    Scabies — 57

Section 3: Emergency — 59
    Shock — 61
    Pulmonary Embolism (PE) — 66

Snakebite	*69*
Nexus Criteria	*75*
Canadian C Spine Rule	*76*
Section 4: Endocrinology	**77**
Type 1 Diabetes Mellitus	*79*
Type 2 Diabetes Mellitus	*82*
Diabetic Ketoacidosis (DKA)	*85*
Thyroid Diseases	*88*
Section 5: Gastroenterology	**93**
Gastroesophageal Reflux Disease (GERD)	*95*
Irritable Bowel Syndrome (IBS)	*97*
Acute Gastroenteritis	*100*
Acute Cholecystitis	*102*
Acute Pancreatitis	*104*
Peptic Ulcer Disease (PUD)	*107*
Diverticulitis	*109*
Hepatic Encephalopathy	*113*
Section 6: Geriatric	**117**
Delirium	*119*
Dementia	*120*
Section 7: Hematology	**123**
Classification of Anemia	*125*
Sickle Cell Anemia	*126*
Multiple Myeloma	*132*
Henoch-Schoenlein Purpura	*137*
Idiopathic Thrombocytopenic Purpura	*139*
Section 8: Infectious Diseases	**141**

Viral Hepatitis	*143*
Pulmonary Tuberculosis	*146*
Influenza	*149*
Dengue Fever	*152*
Tetanus	*155*
Pertussis	*158*
Brucellosis	*160*
Malaria	*162*
Chickenpox	*165*
Infectious Mononucleosis	*167*
Oral Candidiasis	*169*
Fever of Unknown Origin	*171*

Section 9: Musculoskeletal — 173

Acute Low Back Pain	*177*
Osteoarthritis	*179*
Osteoporosis	*182*
Scaphoid Fracture	*185*
Gout	*187*
Fibromyalgia	*190*
Plantar Fasciitis	*192*
Osteomyelitis	*193*
Paronychia	*195*

Section 10: Nephrology — 199

Renal Stone	*201*

Section 11: Neurology — 207

Cerebrovascular Accident (CVA)	*209*
Transient Ischemic Attack (TIA)	*214*

Heatstroke	*218*
Headache	*221*
Multiple Sclerosis	*225*
Febrile Seizure	*229*
Status Epilepticus	*231*
Bell's Palsy	*234*
Benign Paroxysmal Positional Vertigo (BPPV)	*236*
Cervical Dystonia	*239*
Section 12: Obstetrics and Gynecology	**241**
Antenatal Care	*243*
Infertility	*246*
Menopause	*250*
Abnormal Uterine Bleeding (AUB)	*254*
Antepartum Hemorrhage (APH)	*257*
Postpartum Hemorrhage (PPH)	*260*
Folic Acid Supplementation in Pregnancy	*265*
Section 13: Ophthalmology	**267**
Allergic Conjunctivitis	*269*
Infective Conjunctivitis	*271*
Section 14: Otolaryngology	**273**
Acute Otitis Media	*275*
Section 15: Pediatrics	**277**
Acute Epiglottitis	*279*
Transient Synovitis (TS)	*281*
Croup	*283*
Bronchitis	*285*
Bronchiolitis	*287*

Kawasaki Disease	*289*
Scarlet Fever	*291*
Cystic Fibrosis (CF)	*294*
Hand, Foot, and Mouth Disease	*296*
Tetralogy of Fallot	*299*
Coarctation of the Aorta	*301*
Attention Deficit Hyperactivity Disorder (ADHD)	*303*
Encopresis	*306*
Enuresis	*308*
Failure to Thrive (FTT)	*310*
Barlow Maneuver	*312*
Ortolani Maneuver	*313*
Rickets	*314*
Section 16: Respiratory	**317**
Differential Diagnosis of Dyspnea	*319*
Bronchial Asthma	*321*
Chronic Obstructive Pulmonary Disease (COPD)	*325*
Section 17: Urology	**329**
Benign Prostatic Hyperplasia (BPH)	*331*
Section 18: Miscellaneous	**335**
Dehydration and Fluid Management	*337*
Ankle Brachial Index (ABI)	*340*
Hyperkalemia	*341*
Hyponatremia	*345*
Metabolic Syndrome	*350*
Hyperthermia Vs Hyperpyrexia	*352*
Red Man Syndrome	*353*

Insomnia	*355*
Sleep Apnea	*357*
Restless Leg Syndrome (RLS)	*360*
Preoperative Risk Assessment	*362*
Indications of Magnesium Sulfate	*363*
Classifications of Antibiotics	*364*
Mentzer Index	*366*
Antidotes	*367*
Snjad-Sakati Syndrome (SSS)	*369*

Section 1: Cardiovascular

Heart Failure

- Heart failure (HF) is a condition that occurs when the heart cannot pump or fill with enough blood.
- It is a clinical syndrome, resulting from almost any cardiac disorder that impairs the ability of the ventricle to fill with or eject blood.
- It is the end result clinical condition of imbalance between cardiac output and tissue demand.
- The term "heart failure" is misleading because the heart does not completely fail or stop.
- Classifications:

  o Clinically:
    - *Forward*: the heart is unable to maintain adequate cardiac output to meet demand or is able to do so only by elevating filling pressure.
    - *Backward*: the heart is unable to accommodate venous return resulting in elevated filling pressure and vascular congestion (systemic or pulmonary).

  o Anatomically:
    - *Left-sided*: results from diminished peripheral blood pressure and flow.
    - *Right-sided*: usually the consequence of left-sided HF. Isolated right-sided HF is secondary to pulmonary disease.
    - *Biventricular*.

- Physiologically:
    - *Systolic*: inability of the heart to contract effectively.
    - *Diastolic*: impaired filling/relaxation.
- Onset:
    - *Acute*: develops rapidly ((hours/ days).
    - *Chronic*: long-term condition (months/years).
- Hemodynamic:
    - Low-output.
    - High-output.

- Causes:
  - HF is caused by a disease or condition that damages the heart.
  - The most common causes of HF include:
    - *Hypertension*: increase workload of the heart (increase afterload).
    - *Coronary heart disease*: causes narrowing of the blood vessels that supply the heart muscle reducing the flow of blood through vessels low oxygen and ischemia may lead to myocardial infarction (decreased contractility).
    - *Heart valve disease*:
      - The valve can become narrow (stenosed) which interferes with blood flow through the valve and increase pressure in the heart.
      - In other cases, the valve can become leaky (insufficient) causing blood to flow backward (regurgitation).

- *Cardiomyopathy*: heart muscle is damaged leading to enlarged, poorly pumping heart.
- *Chronic anemia*.
- *Hyperthyroidism*.
- *Pregnancy*.

- Pathophysiology:

  o The Frank-Starling mechanism:

    - *Compensated HF*: as cardiac failure progress, end-diastolic pressures increase cardiac muscle fibers stretch increases the volume of the cardiac chamber these lengthened fibers initially contract more forcibly, thereby increasing cardiac output the dilated ventricle is able to maintain cardiac output at a level that meets the needs of the body.
    - *Decompensated HF*: increasing dilation increases ventricle wall tension increases the oxygen requirements the filing myocardium is no longer able to propel sufficient blood to meet the needs of the body, even at rest.

- Clinical features include:

  o Left-sided HF:

    - Fatigue, syncope, systemic hypotension, cool extremities, slow capillary refill, peripheral cyanosis, pulsus alternans, mitral regurgitation, S3 heart sound, dyspnea, orthopnea, PND, cough, crackles, displaced PMI to the left due to cardiomegaly.

- Right-sided HF:
    - The right side of the heart cannot pump efficiently, causing fluid to accumulate in the veins.
    - Tricuspid regurgitation, peripheral edema, JVP, hepatomegaly, ascites, nocturia.

- Diagnosis:
    - Suspect HF in patients with clinical features of heart failure.
    - Identify potential precipitating factors for acute HF including new or worsened left ventricular dysfunction, noncompliance with medications and/or diet, volume overload, drug exposure, arrhythmia, valvular disease, and/or uncontrolled hypertension.
    - Obtain the following initial tests in a patient with suspected HF:
        - ECG.
        - Chest x-ray.
        - Blood tests including CBC, serum chemistries, fasting lipid profile, LFTs, and TSH.
        - BNP or NT-proBNP.
        - Transthoracic echocardiography (TTE) to confirm diagnosis of heart failure with reduced ejection fraction and assess left ventricular ejection fraction.
    - *The New York Heart Association (NYHA) Classification for HF comprises 4 classes, based on the relationship between symptoms and the amouAnt of effort required to provoke them:*

Class	Patient Symptoms (Functional Capacity)
I	No limitation of physical activity
II	Slight limitation of physical activity, comfortable at rest. Ordinary physical activity results in fatigue, palpitations, dyspnea
III	Marked limitation of physical activity, comfortable at rest. Less than ordinary activity causes symptoms.

IV	Unable to carry on any physical activity without discomfort. Symptoms at rest.

- *The American College of Cardiology/American Heart Association (ACC/AHA) HF guidelines complement the NYHA classification to reflect the progression of disease:*

Class	Objective Assessment
A	No objective evidence of CVD. High risk of HF but no structural heart disease
B	Objective evidence of minimal CVD (structural heart disease but no symptoms of HF)
C	Objective evidence of moderately severe CVD. Structural heart disease with symptoms
D	Objective evidence of severe CVD. Severe limitations. Experiences symptoms even at rest. Refractory HF requiring specialized interventions

- The Framingham criteria for the diagnosis of HF consists of the concurrent presence of either 2 major criteria, or 1 major and 2 minor criteria:

Major Criteria	Minor Criteria
Paroxysmal nocturnal dyspnea (PND)	Nocturnal cough
Weight loss of 4.5 kg in 5 days in response to treatment	Dyspnea on ordinary exertion
Neck vein distension	A decreased in vital capacity by one third the maximal value recorded
Rales	Pleural effusion
Acute pulmonary edema	Tachycardia (rate of 120 BPM)
Hepatojugular reflex	Bilateral ankle edema
S3 gallop	

Central venous pressure greater than 16 cm water	
Circulation time of 25 seconds	
Radiographic cardiomegaly	
Pulmonary edema, visceral congestion, or cardiomegaly at autopsy	

- Management:

    o Non-pharmacological (diet and lifestyle):

    - Decrease salt intake < 2 grams per day, decrease fluid < 2 L per day, weight control.

    o For acute heart failure:

    - Administer oxygen in patients with capillary oxygen < 90%.
    - Administer IV loop diuretics (such as furosemide 40-100 mg to treat fluid overload.
    - Use invasive hemodynamic monitoring with pulmonary artery catheter to guide therapy in patients with suspected HF in whom fluid status cannot be determined clinically.
    - Give venous thromboembolism prophylaxis with unfractionated heparin, low-molecular weight heparin, or fondaparinux for those patients being hospitalized unless risk for bleeding outweighs likely benefits (consider IMPROVE Combined Risk Calculator).
    - Continue oral beta blockers and ACEIs or ARBs, or initiate after optimization of volume status and before hospital discharge unless hemodynamically unstable.

    o For selected patients with heart failure with reduced ejection fraction requiring further management:

    - For black patients with persistent symptomatic HF, NYHA class III-IV, prescribe Hydralazine plus Isosorbide dinitrate.

- For patients with symptomatic HF despite treatment with other medications and with serum creatinine < 2.5 mg/dL in men or < 2 mg/dL in women, and potassium < 5 mmol/L, prescribe aldosterone antagonist (such as spironolactone).
- Refer selected patients with stage C HFrEF due to ischemic cardiomyopathy and stage C due to non-ischemic cardiomyopathy for implantable cardioverter-defibrillator (ICD).
- Refer patient for cardiac resynchronization therapy (CRT) if the patient has advanced HF and a QRS interval > 120 milliseconds.

o Inotropes (such as digoxin and amiodarone), indicated in patients with sinus rhythm and symptomatic on ACEIs, or congestive heart failure and AFib.

Hypertension

- Hypertension is a sustained elevation of systemic arterial blood pressure.
- Hypertension is most commonly defined as systolic blood pressure (SBP) ≥ 140 mm Hg or diastolic blood pressure (DBP) ≥ 90 mm Hg, but definitions vary by professional organization.
- Risk factors include:

    o Weight gain.
    o Obesity.
    o Alcohol use (particularly for men).
    o Exposure to insulin.

- Most patients with hypertension have primary or essential hypertension, but in 10%-15% of patients it may be due to secondary causes.
- Evaluation:

    o Initial Diagnosis:

        ▪ Measure blood pressure with the appropriate cuff size in a calm, seated position and with the patient's arm supported at the level of the heart.
        ▪ A hypertension diagnosis is based on ≥ 2 blood pressure measurements per visit, at ≥ 2 visits, with systolic blood pressure (SBP) ≥ 140 mm Hg and/or diastolic blood pressure (DBP) ≥ 90 mm Hg when using manual measurement methods.

    o Confirmation:

        ▪ Blood pressure measurements obtained outside of a clinical setting (ambulatory blood pressure monitoring [ABPM] and home BP monitoring) are recommended for the diagnostic

confirmation of hypertension after the initial screening and before starting treatment.
- Use ABPM if there is diagnostic uncertainty or suspected blood pressure variability.

- Additional Testing:

   - Uniformly recommended testing for all patients with hypertension includes:

     - Blood tests (sodium, potassium, creatinine, fasting glucose, fasting lipid profile).
     - Urine tests (blood, protein).
     - Electrocardiogram (ECG).

- Consider assessment of 10-Year Risk of Cardiovascular Events

- Management:

  - Non-pharmacological Management:

    - Encourage lifestyle modifications which reduce blood pressure and have other health benefits including:

      - Weight reduction if overweight or obese.
      - Dietary changes (decreased fat intake and increased intake of fruits, vegetables, and low-fat dairy).
      - Physical activity.
      - Smoking cessation.

    - Consider sodium restriction and limiting alcohol consumption, but the effects on reducing cardiovascular events or mortality are less certain.

- Pharmacological Management:

    o The decision to start medications for blood pressure lowering should be individualized with shared decision-making including considerations of:

        - The patient's estimated 10-year cardiovascular risk.
        - The estimated risk reduction from medications (considering the patient's baseline risk and systolic blood pressure).
        - The potential adverse effects and burdens of medications used.
        - Any comorbidities or factors affecting risks for cardiovascular events or adverse effects.
        - The patient's values and preferences.

Dyslipidemia

- Dyslipidemias cover a range of lipid abnormalities which may include any combination of:

  o Increased:

    - Total cholesterol (generally ≥ 240 mg/dL [6.2 mmol/L]).
    - Low-density lipoprotein (LDL) cholesterol (generally > 160 mg/dL [4.14 mmol/L]).
    - Triglyceride levels (generally > 200 mg/dL [2.3 mmol/L]).

  o Decreased high-density lipoprotein (HDL) cholesterol levels (generally < 40 mg/dL [1.03 mmol/L]).

- Lipid screening-recommendations for adults differ by professional organization, but screening adults every 4-6 years between the ages of 20 and 79 years is reasonable, with strongest evidence for screening in patients ≥ 40 years old and with certain comorbid conditions
- Management:

Acute Coronary Syndrome

- ACS includes a spectrum of conditions associated with acute myocardial ischemia and/or necrosis usually secondary to reduction in coronary blood flow, including:

    o <u>Unstable angina (UA): also known as Crescendo angina</u>

    - With UA, oxygen demand is unchanged. Supply is decreased secondary to reduced resting coronary flow. This is in contrast to stable angina, which is due to increased demand.
    - Patients usually present with new-onset angina that is severe and worsening, or patients with angina at rest.
    - Cardiac enzymes are NOT elevated.

    o <u>NSTEMI:</u>

    - It's differentiated from UA by the presence of myocardial necrosis.
    - MI is due to necrosis of myocardium as a result of an interruption of blood supply (after a thrombotic occlusion of a coronary artery previously narrowed by athero-sclerosis).
    - Subendocardial (involves inner one-third to one-half of the wall); tends to be smaller.

    o <u>STEMI:</u>

    - It typically occurs when a clot lead to complete occlusion of a coronary artery with trans-mural, or full thickness myocardial infarction.

- The most common cause of ACS is plaque rupture of underlying coronary artery disease (CAD).
- Common risk factors for the ACS include:

    o Smoking, dyslipidemia, HTN, DM, and family history of CAD.

- Clinical features include:

    o Angina in the retrosternal area, occurring at rest or with minimal exertion, and/or hemodynamic instability.

- Workup include:

    o ECG within 10 min. of arrival then repeated at 15-30 minutes if the patient still symptomatic.
    o Measure cardiac troponin I or T in all patients with chest pain consistent with ACS.
    o Perform urgent coronary angiography, unless contraindicated, in patients with non-STEMI with refractory angina, or hemodynamic instability.

- Management:

    o Hospital admission on a floor with continuous cardiac monitoring. Establish IV access and give supplemental oxygen if the patient has arterial saturation < 90% or respiratory distress.
    o Aspirin 162-325 mg (chewed) as soon as possible after presentation.

    - DON'T GIVE NSAIDS EXCEPT ASPIRIN.

    o Add clopidogrel 300 mg the 75 mg once daily as soon as possible.
    o Add anticoagulation therapy (unfractionated heparin, enoxaparin, or bivalirudin) to antiplatelet as soon as possible. Keep PTT at 2 to 2.5 times normal if using unfractionated heparin; PTT NOT followed with LMWH.

- Nitroglycerin 0.3 to 0.4 mg sublingually every 5 minutes for up to 3 doses.
- IV nitroglycerin in the first 48 hours if the patient has persistent ischemia, hart failure, or uncontrolled HTN.
- Beta blocker orally within the first 24 hours unless contraindicated.
- Oral ACEIs (if NO hypotension or contraindications) within the first 24 hours in patients with HTN or left ventricular ejection fraction (LVEF) < 40%.

- Long-term management (in the absence of contraindications) if the patient NOT already taking include:

  - Dual antiplatelet therapy with aspirin, ticagrelor, clopidogrel.
  - Beta blockers.
  - ACE inhibitors.
  - Statin, regardless of lipid levels.
  - Give all patients sublingual or spray nitroglycerin prior to hospital discharge.
  - Continue medication prescribed for secondary prevention.

- Methods of re-vascularization:

  - Percutaneous coronary intervention (PCI):
    - This is the preferred treatment for STEMI.
    - Also preferred in patients with contraindications for thrombolytic therapy; no risk of intracranial hemorrhage.

  - Thrombolytic therapy:
    - It is useful for patients who present later.
    - Administer as soon as possible up to 24 hours after the onset of chest pain.
    - Outcome is best if given within the first 6 hours.
    - Options include Alteplase, Streptokinase, reteplase, and urokinase.

- *Indications*: ST segment elevation in 2 contiguous ECG leads in patients with pain onset within 6 hours who have been refractory to nitroglycerin.
- *Absolute contraindications to thrombolytic therapy*: Trauma, previous stroke, recent invasive procedure or surgery, dissecting aortic aneurysm, active bleeding or bleeding diathesis.

- Coronary artery bypass grafting:
  - Less often used in the acute setting.
  - Benefits include low rates of event free survival and re-intervention free survival.
  - It remains the procedure of choice in patients with severe multi-vessel disease and complex coronary anatomy.

- Complications of acute MI include:
  - Pump failure (CHF).
  - Arrhythmias:
    - Such as Premature ventricular contractions (PVC), A. Fib., and ventricular tachycardia.
  - Recurrent infarction.
  - Mechanical complications.
    - Such as free wall rupture, papillary muscle rupture, and ventricular pseudoaneurysm.
  - Acute pericarditis.
  - Dressler's syndrome (post-myocardial infarction syndrome):
    - Immunologically based syndrome consisting of fever, malaise, pericarditis, leukocytosis, and pleuritis, occurring weeks to months after an MI.

TABLE 1-1 ECG Findings Based on Location of Infarct

Location of Infarct	ECG Changes
Anterior	ST segment elevation in V1–V4 (acute/active)
	Q waves in leads V1–V4 (late change)
Posterior	Large R wave in V1 and V2
	ST segment depression in V1 and V2
	Upright and prominent T waves in V1 and V2
Lateral	Q waves in leads I and aVL (late change)
Inferior	Q waves in leads II, III, aVF (late change)

Note: Augmented ECG leads from aVL indicate the left arm, and from aVF indicate the left foot.

Palpitation

- Palpitations are defined as awareness of a heart beat that may be described by patients as a disagreeable sensation of pulsation or movement in the chest or adjacent areas that may be associated with discomfort, alarm, or pain.
- Differential diagnosis include:

  o Cardiac arrhythmias.

    - Such as ventricular tachycardia, SVT, atrial fibrillation, atrial flutter.

  o Structural heart disease.

    - Such as mitral valve prolapse, mitral or aortic regurgitation, or congenital disease.

  o Psychosomatic disorders.

    - Including anxiety, panic attack, depression, somatization disorders.

  o Systemic conditions.

    - Such as hyperthyroidism, DM, postmenopausal syndrome, anemia, POTS.

  o Medications.

    - Including vasodilators, anticholinergics, hydralazine, recent withdraw of beta blockers.

- o Stimulants and recreational substances.

- Evaluation of patient:

  - o Initial evaluation includes a history and physical exam plus an ECG.

    - Frog sign (prominent JVP) may be present in patients with SVT, especially AVNRT.
    - Termination of palpitation after vagal maneuvers in hemodynamically stable patients, suggests SVT.
    - For wide QRS complex tachycardia, assume ventricular tachycardia until proven otherwise.
    - For regular, narrow QRS tachycardia may suggest sinus tachycardia, atrial flutter, SVT, junctional ectopic tachycardia.
    - Irregular, wide QRS tachycardia may suggest AFib with BBB.
    - Irregular, narrow QRS tachycardia may suggest AFib, atrial flutter.

  - o Consider blood tests in patients with suspected systemic etiology (such as electrolytes or thyroid stimulating hormone to detect hyperthyroidism).
  - o Additional tests may include stress testing, echocardiography, and electrophysiological studies.

- Management:

  - o Provide reassurance for patients with benign palpitations.

    - Reassurance is optimal for patients with benign palpitations, including patients with ventricular premature depolarizations without structural heart disease, ventricular or atrial ectopy, normal sinus rhythm during palpitations.

  - o Psychiatric counseling may be helpful in patients with a recent stressful life event.

- Direct therapy at the etiology in patients with an established cause of palpitations.

    - For acute treatment of regular supraventricular tachycardia of unknown mechanism:

        - Vagal maneuvers and/or IV adenosine are recommended.
        - In hemodynamically unstable patients, synchronized direct current (DC) cardioversion recommended when vagal maneuvers or adenosine ineffective or unfeasible.
        - In hemodynamically stable patients unresponsive to vagal maneuvers and/or IV adenosine, IV diltiazem or verapamil can be effective. IV beta blockers are reasonable.

    - For acute treatment of atrioventricular nodal reentrant tachycardia (AVNRT):

        - Vagal maneuvers and/or IV adenosine are recommended.

    - For acute treatment of atrial tachycardia:

        - IV adenosine can be useful to restore sinus rhythm.
        - IV beta blockers, diltiazem, verapamil can be useful.
        - IV amiodarone may be reasonable to restore rhythm or slow ventricular rate.
        - Indications for hospitalization:

- Hospitalize patients for immediate therapy if imminent risk of serious cardiac arrhythmias, such as patients with:
    - Bradyarrhythmia requiring permanent pacemaker implantation, such as atrioventricular (AV) conduction disorders or sick sinus syndrome.
    - Ventricular tachyarrhythmia or SVT requiring any immediate termination, ICD implantation, or catheter ablation.
    - Symptoms of heart failure (such as dyspnea on exertion) or hemodynamic compromise (such as confusion, chest pain, or syncope).
    - Severe structural heart disease requiring surgery or other procedure.

Atrial Fibrillation

- AF is a common supraventricular tachyarrhythmia caused by uncoordinated atrial activation and associated with an irregularly irregular ventricular response.
- Causes of atrial fibrillation include:

  - Heart disease: CAD, MI, HTN, mitral valve disease.
  - Pericarditis and pericardial trauma (e.g. surgery).
  - Pulmonary disease (including PE).
  - Thyroid diseases.
  - Systemic illnesses (e.g. sepsis, malignancy, DM).
  - Stress (e.g. postoperative).

- Clinical features include:

  - Fatigues, exertional dyspnea, palpitations, dizziness, angina, irregularly irregular pulse.

- Diagnosis:

  - ECG findings: irregularly irregular rhythm (irregular RR intervals and NO identified P waves).

- Management:

  - Acute AFib in a hemodynamically unstable patient:
    - Immediate electrical cardioversion to sinus rhythm.
  - Acute AFib in a hemodynamically stable patient:

- Rate control:

    - If the pulse is too rapid, it must be treated to be between 60 to 100 bpm.
    - Beta blockers are preferred, CCBs are an alternative.
    - If left ventricular systolic dysfunction is present, consider digoxin or amiodarone (useful for rhythm control).

- Cardioversion to sinus rhythm (after rate control is achieved):

    - Candidates for cardioversion include those who are hemodynamically unstable, those with worsening symptoms, and those who are having their first ever AFib.
    - Electrical cardioversion is preferred over pharmacologic cardioversion.
    - Use pharmacologic cardioversion only if electrical cardioversion fails or is not feasible (e.g. Parenteral iblutilide, procainamide, flecainide, sotalol, or amiodarone are choices).

- Anticoagulation to prevent embolic CVA:

    - If AFib present > 48 hours or unknown period of time, risk of embolization during cardioversion is significant (2% to 5%). Anticoagulate patients for 3 weeks before and 4 weeks after cardioversion.
    - An INR of 2 to 3 is the anticoagulation goal range.
    - To avoid waiting 3 weeks for anticoagulation, obtain a transesophageal echocardiogram (TEE) to image the left atrium. If no thrombus is present, start IV heparin and perform cardioversion within 24 hours. Patients still require 4 weeks of anticoagulation after cardioversion.

- Chronic AFib:
    - Rate control with beta blocker or CCB.
    - Anticoagulation:
        - Patients with "lone" AFib (i.e. AFib in the absence of underlying heart disease or other cardioversion risk factors) under age 60 do NOT require anticoagulation because they are at low risk for embolization (aspirin may be appropriate).
        - Treat all other patients with chronic anticoagulation (warfarin).

Giant Cell Arteritis

- Giant cell arteritis is a chronic systemic vasculitis involving large and medium-sized arteries, most commonly the temporal and other cranial arteries.
- It is the most common form of systemic vasculitis affecting persons > 50 years old.
- Temporal arteritis is a medical emergency due to risk of sudden blindness without early detection and treatment.
- 40%-60% of patients with giant cell arteritis have polymyalgia rheumatic (PMR) symptoms, while 15% of patients with PMR will develop giant cell vasculitis.
- Clinical features include:

    o Temporal arteritis is typically characterized by abrupt onset of a unilateral continuous headache and/or pain in the temporal region that is unresponsive to analgesia.
    o Other characteristic symptoms include pain on chewing or swallowing, tongue pain, scalp tenderness, and/or ocular involvement which can include amaurosis fugax (transient blindness), blurry vision, or double vision.
    o Other presentations of giant cell arteritis may include constitutional symptoms, myalgia and stiffness of the neck and the hip and/or shoulder girdle, limb claudication, and neuropathies.

- Diagnosis:

    o There are no universally accepted diagnostic criteria for giant cell arteritis, but the American College of Rheumatology (ACR) provisional classification criteria require at least 3 of the following: age > 50 years, localized headache that was not preexisting, temporal

    artery tenderness or reduced pulsation, elevated ESR > 50 mm/hour, and abnormal arterial biopsy.
  - Diagnose patients with temporal arteritis who have the appropriate clinical presentation and response to steroid therapy, even if the temporal artery biopsy results are negative.
  - For suspected large-vessel giant cell arteritis, obtain imaging with positron emission tomography (PET) or MRI for diagnosis.

- Management:

  - Initial corticosteroid therapy (1 mg/kg body weight orally/day, maximum daily dose 60 mg) as soon as clinical diagnosis of temporal arteritis is made.
  - Do not delay by waiting to confirm diagnosis by biopsy or imaging.
  - Consider initial treatment of methylprednisolone 250-1000 mg/day IV for 3-5 days, and then transition to oral dosing for patients with cerebral or ocular symptoms or to allow more rapid tapering.

Chads$_2$ Score

- The score is a clinical prediction for estimating the risk of stroke in patients with non-valvular AFib.

Score	CHADS$_2$ Risk Criteria
1 point	Congestive heart failure
1 point	Hypertension
1 point	Age > 75 years
1 point	Diabetes Mellitus
2 points	Stroke / TIA

CHADS$_2$ Score	Risk	Recommendation
0	Low	Aspirin 81-325 mg daily
1	Intermediate	Aspirin daily or warfarin
2 or more	High	Warfarin unless contraindicated

Has-Bled Score

- It is a scoring system developed to assess 1-year risk of major bleeding in patients with AFib.

Clinical Characteristic	Point
Hypertension	1 point
Abnormal liver function	1 point
Abnormal renal function	1 point
Stroke	1 point
Bleeding	1 point
Labile INRs	1 point
Elderly (Age > 65)	1 point
Drugs predisposing to bleeding	1 point
Alcohol	1 point

Score	Bleeding risk classification (% bleeds per 100 patient-years)
0-1	Low risk (1.1%)
2	Intermediate risk (1.9%)
> 3	High risk (4.9%)

NOAC Anticoagulation

- The Novel Oral Anticoagulants (NOACs) are a new class of anticoagulant drug.
- They can be used in the prevention of stroke for people with non-valvular AFib, or in the management of venous thromboembolism (VTE).
- Examples include Dabigatran, Rivaroxaban, and Apixaban.
- All of the NOACs have been shown to be as effective at preventing strokes as warfarin. The main difference between NOACs and warfarin is that NOACs are less influenced by diet and other medications.
- If a person has a high risk of bleeding, then oral anticoagulation, including NOACs and warfarin, may not be recommended.
- The main obstacle is that NOACs are more expensive than warfarin.

Pulseless Electrical Activity (PEA)

- PEA, also known as electromechanical dissociation, is a common cause of cardiopulmonary arrest in the hospital setting.
- PEA refers to cardiac arrest in which the ECG shows a heart rhythm that should produce a pulse, but does not.
- Etiologies of PEA that are potentially treatable include hypovolemia, hypoxia, hyperkalemia, sever acidosis, pulmonary embolism, cardiac tamponade, and tension pneumothorax.
- The loss of cardiac output results from decreased ventricular filling (hypovolemia, PE, cardiac tamponade, or tension pneumothorax) or electromechanical dissociation (hypoxia, hyperkalemia, or severe acidosis).
- Physical examination focuses of potential correctable etiologies.
- Management of PEA arrest requires rapid establishment of vascular access, airway stabilization, and administration of IV fluids.

    o Rapid saline bolus is more likely to be effective and can be given immediately.

- If sepsis is suspected, broad-spectrum antibiotics would be appropriate, but antibiotic administration will not affect the immediate outcome of the cardiopulmonary arrest.
- Electrical cardioversion will not benefit a patient in sinus rhythm. Similarly, cardiac pacing will not help, since the problem is not associated with severe bradycardia.

Section 2: Dermatology

Acne Vulgaris

- Acne is a chronic skin condition characterized by non-inflammatory open and/or closed comedones (blackheads and whiteheads) and inflammatory lesions (papules, pustules, cysts or nodules) typically located on the face, neck, back, chest, and upper arms.
- Comedones develop when excess sebum production due to androgen excess blocks hair follicles. The proliferation of *Propionibacterium acnes* on the skin contributes to inflammatory lesions.
- Risk factors:

    o Acne is most common at ages 16-20 years.
    o Acne is more common and more severe in males at puberty.
    o Drugs that may produce acne or acneiform eruptions include anabolic steroids and antiepileptic drugs.
    o Factors that may contribute to flares or worsening of acne include:

    - Menstrual cycle, Picking, Emotional stress, Occlusion of skin surface with greasy products, Sweating, Pregnancy.

- Causes:

    o Androgen production (usually occurs at puberty) stimulates sebaceous gland to increases sebum production.

    - Hyperproliferation and shedding of keratinocytes in clumps blocks outflow of sebum from hair follicle, forming a comedone.

    o Medications associated with onset or exacerbation of acne may include isoniazid, phenytoin, cyclosporine, vitamins B1, B2, B6, B12, and D2.

- Clinical features:

    - The chief complaint usually are acne, pimples, or skin blemishes.

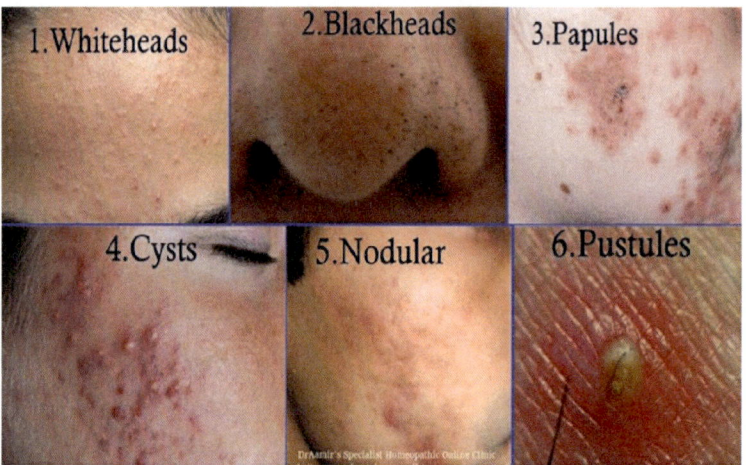

- Diagnosis:

    - Diagnosis is made by physical exam.
    - Clinical evaluation is used to consider secondary or associated conditions.

- Classifications:

    - *Mild*: if scattered open and/or closed comedones are the predominant lesion type, with few inflammatory lesions.
    - *Moderate*: if superficial inflammatory lesions (papulopustular or polymorphic) predominate with some comedones.
    - *Severe*: if there are numerous large papules and/or pustules and/or multiple nodules (nodulocystic) and deep lesions, evidence of scarring, and/or involvement of large areas.

- Non-pharmacological management include:

    - Advise the patient that acne is not associated with poor hygiene.
    - Improvement may take up to 4-8 weeks following treatment.

- o Acne or skin irritation may appear to worsen during early treatment with certain medications (particularly retinoids).

- Pharmacological management include:

  - o First-line therapy in non-pregnant patients with mild acne:

    - Offer monotherapy with topical retinoid, preferred if comedonal acne, or benzoyl peroxide.
    - Or offer combination therapy, particularly if the patient has mixed inflammatory and non-inflammatory lesions, with benzoyl peroxide plus topical clindamycin.
    - Or offer triple topical therapy with a retinoid, clindamycin, and benzoyl peroxide.

  - o For moderate acne and acne unresponsive to topical therapy, in non-pregnant patients aged > 8 years:

    - Add oral antibiotic to topical combination therapy of topical retinoid plus benzoyl peroxide.
    - Consider Doxycycline with dosing for acne for adults and children aged > 8 years and > 100 pounds, as 50-100 mg once or twice daily.
    - To reduce potential for bacterial resistance, do not use topical antibiotics or oral antibiotics as monotherapy, but combine with topical benzoyl peroxide, and consider limiting duration of oral antibiotic use to 3 months.

  - o For severe acne, or acne resistant to 3 months oral antibiotic plus topical therapy:

    - For women, consider adding combined oral contraceptives or consider oral spironolactone.
    - Or, for men or women, start oral isotretinoin with conventional dosing or low-dose, and prevention against the

possibility of pregnancy while taking isotretinoin, including monthly pregnancy testing for women.
- Check baseline LFT, serum cholesterol, and consider monitoring for depression while on isotretinoin.
- Discontinue oral tetracycline antibiotics while on isotretinoin.

Atopic Dermatitis

- Atopic dermatitis is a chronic, relapsing, inflammatory skin disease affecting primarily children.
- Genetic, dietary, environmental, and infectious factors promote the condition and may trigger relapses and exacerbations.
- It is associated with asthma, allergic rhinitis, food allergy, and Wiskott-Aldrich syndrome.
- Clinical Features and Diagnosis:

  o Diagnosis is based on history and physical findings. Atopic dermatitis often presents as an itchy, erythematous rash but with characteristic locations and patterns found in particular age groups:

    - In infants, atopic dermatitis most often affects the cheeks, chin, scalp, and extensor surfaces of extremities.
    - In older children and adults, the flexor surfaces, neck, wrists, and ankles may be affected.

  o Testing is not necessary unless the patient is not responding to therapy or there is significant diagnostic uncertainty.

- Management:

  o Avoid food or environmental triggers or irritants if clear clinical reaction after exposure to the suspected trigger, and positive allergy testing, if available.
  o Use emollients (moisturizers), including application soon after bathing.
  o Use topical steroids on flaring areas:

- Use low potency for mild symptoms, and for eczema on face and neck. Consider desonide 0.05% gel, cream or ointment, or foam; or fluocinolone 0.01% cream BID.
- Use medium potency, such as for moderate to severe symptoms. Consider betamethasone valerate 0.1% cream or lotion; or fluticasone propionate 0.05% cream twice daily for moderate atopic dermatitis.
- In patients with recurrent flares, use topical steroids once or twice weekly at sites of prior dermatitis, for proactive, maintenance therapy.

- Use topical calcineurin inhibitors (such as tacrolimus 0.1% or pimecrolimus 1% BID) for Recalcitrance to steroids, Sensitive areas (face, anogenital, skin folds) Steroid-induced atrophy, and Long-term uninterrupted topical steroid use.
- Consider UV light therapy or 5-methoxypsoralen + UV A (PUVA) after failure of previous Rx.
- Consider cyclosporine or azathioprine in severe, refractory atopic dermatitis.
- Consider dupilumab in severe, refractory atopic dermatitis.
- Consider bleach baths and intranasal mupirocin if there are signs of secondary bacterial infection.
- Don't recommend dietary exclusions unless confirmed IgE-mediated food allergy.

Contact Dermatitis

- Contact dermatitis is an erythematous, pruritic skin reaction caused by contact with exogenous agents.
- Allergic contact dermatitis is due to a delayed immunologic response (type IV hypersensitivity) to a cutaneous or systemic exposure to an allergen to which the patient has been previously sensitized.

    o There is a latency period of 12-48 hours between exposure to allergen and clinical dermatitis in sensitized patients.
    o Poison ivy, poison sumac, and poison oak (Toxicodendron genus) are the most common causes of allergic (cell-mediated) contact dermatitis in the United States.
    o Nickel is the most common cause of metal dermatitis and most common cause of allergic contact dermatitis worldwide.

- Irritant contact dermatitis is a nonimmunologic reaction to substance or action producing direct damage to skin by chemical abrasion or physical irritation. Causes of irritant contact dermatitis include chemical agents, alcohol, creams, powders, moisture, friction, and temperature extremes.
- Most causes of occupational contact dermatitis are from irritants encountered in the workplace.
- Clinical Features and Diagnosis:

    o Rash typically is a popular or papulovesicular pruritic eruption which may be linear or geometric corresponding to the area of contact.
    o Patients may also present with a disseminated (id reaction) skin eruption if previously sensitized topically and then re-exposed systemically.
    o Allergic dermatitis develops over hours to days whereas irritant dermatitis develops over minutes to hours.

- Diagnosis is usually made clinically, based on history of exposure and localized rash with typical features.
- Testing is not usually needed, but use patch testing to diagnose allergic contact dermatitis and identify contact dermatitis.

- Management:

  - Identify an avoid precipitating the allergen or irritant.
  - When treating contact dermatitis:

    - Use topical corticosteroids for localized or mild-to-moderate contact dermatitis.

- Apply twice daily and continue for 2 weeks.
- Limit higher-potency steroids to use on the extremities and torso.

  - Consider systemic corticosteroids for allergic contact dermatitis that is severe, widespread, or involves the face or mucous membranes.

    - Consider prednisone 40 mg/day orally for 5 days.

  - Consider skin moisturizers to decrease irritation in irritant contact dermatitis.

Scabies

- Scabies is highly contagious, pruritic ectoparasitic infestation of the skin.
- The incubation period for scabies is 7-27 days.
- Mites are transmitted by close extended person-to-person contact and are less commonly transmitted from infested sheets or clothing although they can survive up to 36 hours off of human skin.
- Types:

    o Common scabies:

    - Significant pruritus, especially at night.

    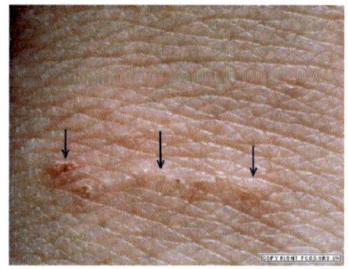

    o Crusted scabies (Norwegian):

    - Pruritus may be mild or absent.

    o Nodular scabies:

    - Persistent pruritic nodules.

- Evaluation:

    o Scabies is a clinical diagnosis based on history and intense pruritus and visible lesions in a typical location (interweb spaces and intertriginous areas).
    o Examination of the patient should be performed with gloves and skin-to-skin contact should be avoided.

- Lesion may include burrows which are linear or wavy and are most commonly located on inter-digital web spaces, flexor wrists, axillae, areolae, umbilicus, genitals, knees, and ankle.
- The burrow ink test, which may help identify a burrow, involves rubbing a scabietic papule with a felt tip or fountain pen, wiping off the ink with alcohol, and looking for linear or zig-zag tracking of the ink along the lesion (tracking suggests the presence of a burrow).
- Topical tetracycline or fluorescein dye applied to a lesion will cause burrows to fluoresce with a Wood's lamp.
- The head/face only tends to be affected in infants; all other ages tend to be affected from the neck down.

- Management:

  - Non-pharmacological treatment includes washing clothing and bedding. Children should be excluded from school until treated.
  - Topical permethrin 5% is the treatment of choice. It should be provided to the patient and to all household/close contacts > 2 months old (even if they are asymptomatic) and should be applied to all skin surfaces from the neck to toes for 8-14 hours and then washed off.
  - Topical Lindane 1% for patients > 2 years old who cannot tolerate permethrin or who failed a first-line therapy, but it carries the risk of neurotoxicity.
  - Topical crotamiton 10% cream or lotion can be used in infants and is applied from the neck down for 2 consecutive nights and then washed off 48 hours after the second application.
  - Oral ivermectin 200 mcg/kg (with a repeat dose at 2 weeks) for patients > 5 years who are not pregnant or lactating.

- Crusted scabies (Norwegian scabies) is difficult to treat. The CDC recommends ivermectin 200 mcg/kg orally on days 1, 2, 8, 9, and 15 (with additional doses on days 22 and 29 for severe cases) in combination with topical permethrin or benzyl benzoate 5% full body application daily for 7 days then twice weekly until cure.
- Symptoms and lesions may persist for up to 1-2 months after treatment.

Section 3: Emergency

Shock

- Shock is an abnormality of the circulatory system that results in inadequate organ perfusion and tissue oxygenation.
- Shock in a trauma patient is classified as hemorrhagic or non-hemorrhagic:

  o Hemorrhagic shock:

    - Hemorrhage is the most common cause of shock after injury, and virtually all patients with multiple injuries have an element of hypovolemia.
    - The primary focus in hemorrhagic shock is to promptly identify and stop hemorrhage.

  o Nonhemorrhagic shock:

    - Cardiogenic shock:

- Myocardial dysfunction can be caused by blunt cardiac injury, cardiac tamponade, an air embolus, or, rarely, a myocardial infarction associated with the patient's injury.

    - Distributive shock:

- Neurogenic shock:

  o Cervical or upper thoracic spinal cord injury can produce hypotension due to loss of sympathetic tone.

- Septic shock:

- o Septic shock can occur in patients with penetrating abdominal injuries and contamination of the peritoneal cavity by intestinal contents.

- Anaphylactic shock:

  - o Caused by a severe anaphylactic reaction to an allergen, antigen, drug or foreign protein causing the release of histamine which causes widespread vasodilation, leading to hypotension and increased capillary permeability.

    - Obstructive shock (is due to obstruction of blood flow outside of the heart):

      - Cardiac tamponade.
      - Tension pneumothorax.
      - Pulmonary embolism.
      - Aortic stenosis.
      - Clinical features include:

- o In most cases, tachycardia is the earliest measurable circulatory sign of shock.
- o Tachycardia is diagnosed when the heart rate is greater than 160 beats per minutes (BPM) in an infant, 140 BPM in a pre-school aged child, 120 BPM in children from school age to puberty, and 100 BPM in adults.
- o Patients with sepsis who also have hypotension and are afebrile are clinically difficult to distinguish from those in hypovolemic shock, as both groups can manifest tachycardia, cutaneous vasoconstriction, impaired urinary output, decreased systolic pressure, and narrow pulse pressure.
- o Patients with early septic shock can have a normal circulating volume, modest tachycardia, warm skin, systolic pressure near normal, and a wide pulse pressure.

- o Tachycardia, muffled heart sounds, and dilated, engorged neck veins with hypotension resistant to fluid therapy suggest cardiac tamponade.
- o The presence of acute respiratory distress, subcutaneous emphysema, absence breath sounds, hyperresonance to percussion, and tracheal shift supports the diagnosis of tension pneumothorax.
- o The classic picture of neurogenic shock is hypotension without tachycardia or cutaneous vasoconstriction. A narrowed pulse pressure is not seen in neurogenic shock.
- o Anaphylactic reactions typically begin within 15 minutes of exposure to the allergen. Anaphylaxis is likely when all of the following 3 criteria are met:

    - Rapid onset and progression of symptoms.
    - Life threatening compromise of one or more of (Airway, Breathing, Circulation).
    - Involvement of skin (erythema, warmness) and/or mucosa (angioedema, GI symptoms).

- Diagnosis:

  - o NO vital sign and no laboratory test can diagnose shock; rather, the initial diagnosis is based on clinical recognition of the presence of inadequate tissue perfusion and oxygenation.
  - o Reliance solely on systolic BP as an indicator of shock can result in delayed recognition of the shock state.
  - o Compensatory mechanisms can preclude a measurable fall in systolic pressure until up to 30% of the patient's blood volume is lost.
  - o The classification of hemorrhage into 4 classes based on clinical signs is a useful tool for estimating the percentage of acute blood loss:

	Class I	Class II	Class III	Class IV
Blood loss (mL)	Up to 750	750-1500	1500-2000	> 2000
Blood loss (%)	Up to 15%	15-30%	30-40%	> 40%
Pulse rate	< 100	100-120	120-140	> 140
Systolic BP	Normal	Normal	Decreased	Decreased
Pulse pressure	Normal or increased	Decreased	Decreased	Decreased
Respirator rate	14-20	20-30	30-40	> 35
Urine output (mL/Hr.)	> 30	20-30	5-15	Negligible
CNS/mental status	Slightly anxious	Mildly anxious	Anxious, confused	Confused, lethargic
Initial fluid replacement	Crystalloid	Crystalloid	Crystalloid and blood	Crystalloid and blood

- Management:

    o Patient treatment is directed toward reversing the shock state by providing adequate oxygenation, ventilation, and appropriate fluid resuscitation, as well as stopping the bleeding if present.
    o Establish 2 large-caliber (minimum of 16-gauge in an adult) peripheral IV catheters.

        ▪ The most desirable sites for peripheral, percutaneous IV lines in adults are the forearms and antecubital veins.

    o Ana initial, warmed fluid bolus is given. The usual dose is 1 to 2 L for adults and 20 mL/kg for pediatric patients.

- Patients who are transient responders or non-responders (those with class III or IV hemorrhage) will need pRBCs and blood products as an early part of their resuscitation.
- Specific management:

    - Cardiac tamponade is best managed by thoracotomy. Pericardiocentesis may be used as a temporizing maneuver when thoracotomy is not an available option.
    - Tension pneumothorax is treated with immediate thoracic decompression without waiting for x-ray confirmation of the diagnosis.
    - Anaphylaxis is treated with 0.5 mL of 1:1000 epinephrine SC, IM if less severe to lateral thigh or IV (1:10,000) if severe. "0.01 mL/kg up to 0.4 mL for children".

Pulmonary Embolism (PE)

- PE represents a mechanical obstruction of one or more branches of the pulmonary vasculature (via the RV and pulmonary artery), usually due to a blood clot (thromboembolism) from DVT.
- Risk factors for DVT/ PE include:

    o Age > 65 years.
    o Malignancy.
    o Prior history of DVT, PE.
    o Hereditary hypercoagulable states (factor V Leiden, protein C and S deficiency, antithrombin III deficiency).
    o Prolonged immobilization or bed rest, long-distance travel.
    o Cardiac disease, especially CHF.
    o Obesity.
    o Nephrotic syndrome.
    o Major surgery, especially pelvic surgery (orthopedic procedures).
    o Major trauma.
    o Pregnancy, estrogen use (oral contraceptives).

- Clinical features include:

    o Dyspnea, tachypnea, tachycardia, pleuritic chest pain, cough, hemoptysis, fever, rales, S4, decreased breath sound, dullness on percussion.

- Diagnosis:

    o Intraluminal filling defects in central, segmental, or lobular pulmonary arteries on helical CT and clinical suspicion.
    o DVT diagnosed with ultrasound and clinical suspicion.
    o Positive pulmonary angiogram (definitely proves PE).

Clinical characteristic	Score	Interpretation
Symptoms of DVT	3 points	Score > 6: high probability
No alternative diagnosis better explains the illness	3 points	
Tachycardia with pulse > 100	1.5 points	Score > 2 and < 6: moderate
Immobilization > 3 days, or surgery in the previous 4 weeks	1.5 points	Score < 2: low probability
Prior history of DVT or PE	1.5 points	
Presence of hemoptysis	1 point	
Presence of malignancy	1 point	

- Management:

    o Supplemental oxygen to correct hypoxemia.
    o Acute anticoagulation therapy with either unfractionated or low-molecular-weight heparin to prevent another PE. Anticoagulation prevents further clot formation, but does not lyse existing emboli or diminish thrombus size.

        ▪ Start immediately on a basis of clinical suspicion.
        ▪ Give one bolus, followed by a continuous infusion for 5 to 10 days.
        ▪ Heparin acts by promoting the action of antithrombin III.

- Contraindications to heparin include active bleeding, uncontrolled HTN, recent stroke, and heparin-induced thrombocytopenia (HIT).

○ Oral warfarin for long-term treatment:

- Can start with heparin on day 1.
- Therapeutic INR is 2 to 3.
- Continue for 3 to 6 months or more, depending on risk factors.

○ Thrombolytic therapy (e.g. streptokinase, TPA).

- Speeds up the lysis of clots.

○ Inferior vena cava interruption (IVC filter placement):

- Indications include:
  - Contraindication to anticoagulation.
  - A complication of current anticoagulation.
  - A patient with low pulmonary reserve who is at high risk for death from PE.
  - Complications of PE include:

○ Arrhythmia.
○ Chronic thromboembolic pulmonary hypertension.
○ Cor pulmonale, which may lead to obstructive shock.

Snakebite

- Snakebites are injuries caused by the bite of a snake that may or may not involve envenomation.
- Risk factors include:

  o Men aged 17-27 years.
  o Occupations associated with increased risk (due to increased frequency of contact) include:

    - Farming (especially rice).
    - Plantation work (for example, rubber and coffee).
    - Herding, hunting, fishing, fish farming.
    - Snake handling (for example, snake charming, food preparation in restaurants that serve snake, sea-snake hunting).

- Factors associated with increased risk of adverse or fatal outcomes following snakebite include:

  o Bites in children (due to higher dose of venom relative to body weight) or elderly patients (due to increased risk for hypotension, therapeutic fluid overload, adverse effects of adrenaline, and existing comorbidities).
  o Inadequate dose of antivenom or use of monospecific antivenom of inappropriate specificity.
  o Delay in hospital treatment.
  o Inadequate ventilator support.
  o Failure to treat hypovolemia in shocked patients.
  o Aspiration, airway obstruction, or respiratory failure due to respiratory paralysis.
  o Complicating infection.

- Inadequate observation of patients after hospital admission.

- Clinical features include:

  - Confirmation and type of envenomation are often determined by the clinical features, circumstantial history of bite, and knowledge of local snakes.
  - Early indications of severe envenoming include:

    - Snake identified as clinically important.
    - Rapid early expansion of local swelling from bite site.
    - Tender lymph node enlargement (indicates spread of venom) within 30-60 minutes.
    - Early systemic symptoms (hypotension, shock, nausea, vomiting, diarrhea, severe headache, "heavy" eyelids, pathologic drowsiness, ptosis).
    - Spontaneous bleeding.
    - Dark brown or black urine.

  - Systemic envenomation is suggested by:

    - Neurotoxic signs and symptoms.
    - Bleeding and clotting disorders.
    - Cardiovascular signs such as hypotension, shock, cardiac arrhythmia, or abnormal ECG.

  - With non-venomous bite, signs and symptoms of terror and anxiety can mimic systemic envenomation.

- Diagnosis and workup:

  - Blood tests for evidence of hemorrhagic envenoming.

    - Testing should include hemostasis testing, CBC, serum biochemical testing, and peripheral smear/blood film to look for schistocytes and other evidence of hemolysis.

- All cases of suspected or confirmed snakebite should be observed with serial blood testing for at least 12 hours to exclude severe envenoming.

  o Urine studies for signs of hemorrhagic envenoming and/or rhabdomyolysis.
  o The snake venom detection kit can help determine the appropriate antivenom in patients with known envenomation from 1 of the 5 major snake groups, but cannot confirm or rule out systemic envenomation.
  o Arterial oxygenation testing for evidence of acidemia (respiratory or metabolic acidosis) or respiratory failure (neurotoxic envenoming).
  o ECG to assess for hyperkalemia.
  o In pregnant women, fetal monitoring to assess for fetal bradycardia.

- Management:

  o Initial treatment include:

    - Immobilize the affected limb with a splint or sling and limit the patient's movement to help prevent systemic absorption of venom.
    - Perform rapid clinical assessment with resuscitation if needed.

  o Harmful treatments that should be avoided include:

    - Cauterization, incision or excision, tattooing or immediate prophylactic amputation of the bitten digit.
    - Suction of venom by mouth or vacuum pumps.
    - Application of ice pack.

  o Tourniquet use is not recommended.

- If used, give antivenom if indicated before loosening tourniquet to reduce the risk of severe envenomation.
- Admit all patients with confirmed or probable snakebite for at least 12-24 hours.
- For intense local pain, oral acetaminophen is preferable to aspirin or NSAIDs to minimize the risk of gastric bleeding in patients with incoagulable blood.
- Treat severe pain with opiates, but monitor for respiratory depression.
- For snakebite with no evidence of envenomation, observe the patient for at least 12 hours and give analgesics as needed.
- Reserve antivenom for patients with signs or symptoms suggestive of systemic or severe local envenomation.
- In patients with a high risk of strong adverse reactions to antivenom:
  - Give antivenom only if there are signs of systemic envenoming.
  - Prepare a prophylactic epinephrine injection, IV antihistamines (both anti-H1, such as promethazine or chlorphenamine and anti-H2, such as cimetidine or ranitidine), and a corticosteroid as a precaution against a reaction to the antivenom before the antivenom is given.
  - Prophylactic epinephrine 250 mcg SC reduces the risk of acute severe adverse reaction to antivenom.
- Always give antivenom IV if possible; with closely monitor patients during and for 2 hours after administration to look for an adverse reaction.
- Specific antivenom selection is based on either snake identification or clinical manifestations and geographic location.
- If the snake species is unidentified, consider using a polyvalent antivenom.
- For patients who are admitted and treated with antivenom, repeat lab studies as an outpatient (CBC, PT/INR, and fibrinogen) every 2-3 days and every 5-7 days following last antivenom dose.

- o Instruct patients to avoid contact sports, dental extractions, tattoos/piercings, and elective surgery for > 2 weeks.

- Antivenom includes:

  - o Crotalidae polyvalent immune fab (CroFab).

    - Start with 4-6 vials/dose IV infused over 1 hr.; monitor for 1 hr. following infusions for allergic reaction; repeat with additional 4-6 vials if control not achieved with initial dose.
    - Once control achieved, may need to administer 2 vials IV q6hr for up to 18 hr.

- Wilderness Medical Society definitions of envenomation severity:

  - o Dry bite includes bites with no local or systemic signs of envenomation after > 8 hours of monitoring.
  - o Minor envenomation includes bites with non-progressive symptoms and no systemic signs.
  - o Moderate envenomation includes bites with:

    - Severe local pain.
    - Worsening edema.
    - Mild-to-moderate systemic symptoms that are not life-threatening.
    - Abnormal coagulation tests.
    - No signs of bleeding.

  - o Severe envenomation includes bites with:

    - Severe swelling and pain.
    - Systemic symptoms that are life-threatening.
    - Abnormal coagulation tests.
    - Serious bleeding.
    - Other common signs or symptoms such as:

- ❖ Hypotension.
- ❖ Systemic bleeding.
- ❖ Neurotoxicity and myotoxicity signs:

  - ➢ Oral paresthesia.
  - ➢ Muscle fasciculations.
  - ➢ Altered mental status.
  - ➢ Seizures.

Nexus Criteria

- National Emergency X-Radiography Utilization Study (NEXUS) Criteria.
- It is used to clear patients from cervical spine fracture clinically without imaging.
- The criteria are:

  o No posterior midline cervical-spine tenderness.

    - If there is pain on palpation of the posterior midline from the nuchal ridge to the prominence of the first thoracic vertebra.

  o No evidence of intoxication.

    - Evidence of intoxication such as an odor of alcohol, slurred speech, ataxia, or dysmetria.

  o Normal level of alertness.

    - An altered level of alertness is GCS of 14 or less, disorientation to person, place time, or events, or inability to remember 3 objects at five minutes.

  o No focal neurological deficit (numbness of weakness).
  o No painful distracting injuries (long bones fractures such as femur).

- Absence of these 5 items indicates NO radiography.
- Any of these 5 items requires radiography.

Canadian C Spine Rule

- The Canadian C-Spine rule is a decision making tool used to determine when radiography should be utilized in patients following trauma.
- It is applicable to patients who are in an alert (GCS of 15) and stable condition following trauma where cervical spine injury is a concern.
- It is not applicable in non-trauma cases, if the patient has unstable vital signs, acute paralysis, known vertebral disease or previous history of cervical spine surgery and age < 16 years.

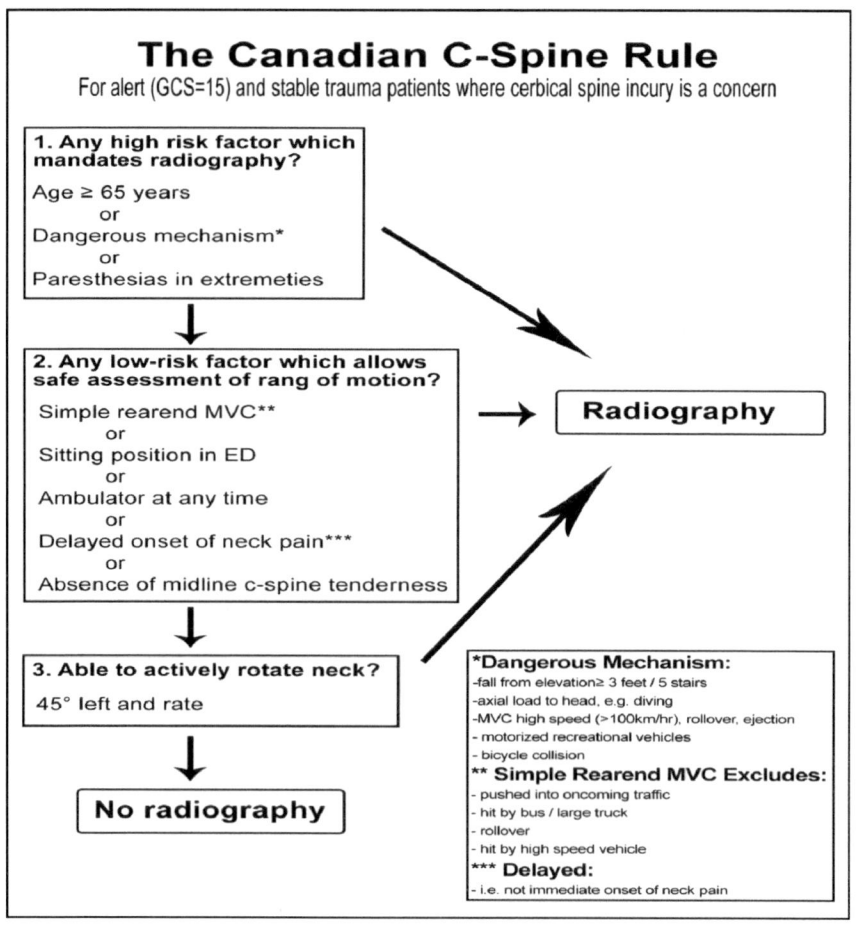

Section 4: Endocrinology

Type 1 Diabetes Mellitus

- Diabetes Mellitus (DM) type 1 is an endocrine disorder characterized by insulin deficiency usually due to autoimmune pancreatic beta-cell destruction, and resulting in hyperglycemia and complications such as ketoacidosis, cardiovascular disease, nephropathy, and retinopathy.
- Type 1 diabetes can occur at any age, but commonly presents in childhood or adolescence, often with classic symptoms such as polyuria, polydipsia polyphagia, and sudden weight loss; about 30% of children and adolescents present in diabetic ketoacidosis (DKA), a metabolic emergency.
- Patients with type 1 diabetes are at increased risk for a number of other immune-mediated disorders, especially autoimmune thyroid disease and celiac disease.
- Evaluation:
    - Perform blood testing to diagnose diabetes:
        - Diagnostic criteria for diabetes is any of the following:
- Fasting plasma glucose ≥ 126 mg/dL (7 mmol/L) (after no caloric intake for ≥ 8 hours).
- Symptoms of hyperglycemia with random plasma glucose ≥ 200 mg/dL (11.1 mmol/L).
- 2-hour plasma glucose ≥ 200 mg/dL (11.1 mmol/L) during a 75-g oral glucose tolerance test.
- HbA1c ≥ 6.5% (HbA1c may not be accurate for diagnosis in cases of pregnancy, hemoglobinopathy, certain anemias, or abnormal erythrocyte loss or replacement).
        - Repeat testing for confirmation in the absence of unequivocal hyperglycemia.

- If diabetic ketoacidosis is suspected, also measure electrolytes, blood urea nitrogen (BUN), creatinine, arterial blood gas, and serum and urine ketones. Urine ketones can be used when serum ketones are not available, but they are reported to have lower sensitivity and specificity compared to serum ketones.
- At least annually, assess urinary albumin (such as spot urinary albumin-to-creatinine ratio) and estimated glomerular filtration rate (GFR) in patients with type 1 diabetes beginning at 5 years after diagnosis to screen for chronic kidney disease.

- Management:

  - All patients with type 1 diabetes require insulin. For most patients, prescribe multiple daily insulin injections (1-2 injections of basal insulin and ≥ 3 injections/day of prandial insulin) or continuous subcutaneous insulin infusion (CSII) (insulin pump).
  - Consider individualized glycemic goals. Generally recommended targets in type 1 diabetes are:
  - HbA1c < 7% in most nonpregnant adults, < 6% in pregnant women, and < 7% across all pediatric age groups.
  - In nonpregnant adults, pre-prandial plasma glucose of 80-130 mg/dL (4.4-7.2 mmol/L) and peak postprandial glucose < 180 mg/dL (10 mmol/L).
  - In pregnancy, fasting glucose < 95 mg/dL (5.3 mmol/L), and either:

    - 1-hour postprandial glucose < 140 mg/dL (7.8 mmol/L).
    - 2-hour postprandial glucose < 120 mg/dL (6.7 mmol/L).

  - Provide support for diabetes self-management education (DSME), including nutritional management.
  - Other medications include:

    - Statins are the medication of choice for lowering low-density lipoprotein cholesterol:

- Prescribe a statin for most adults > 40 years old with diabetes, and consider prescribing a statin if the patient is < 40 years old with cardiovascular risk factors.
- Consider prescribing a statin for children > 10 years old with type 1 diabetes and low-density lipoprotein cholesterol > 160 mg/dL (4.1 mmol/L), or low-density lipoprotein cholesterol > 130 mg/dL (3.4 mmol/L) with ≥ 1 additional cardiovascular risk factor.
- For females of reproductive age, reproductive counseling is suggested prior to initiating a statin due to potential teratogenic effects.

- Offer an angiotensin-converting enzyme (ACE) inhibitor or angiotensin receptor blocker (ARB) in nonpregnant patients with hypertension or albuminuria.
- Consider aspirin 75-162 mg/day for patients with increased cardiovascular risk, after a comprehensive discussion with the patient and if benefits are deemed to outweigh the risk of bleeding.

o For treatment of hypoglycemia:

- Give glucose 15-20 g (or any carbohydrate that contains glucose) orally to a conscious individual, or glucagon if the patient is unconscious or unable to take glucose orally.
- Prescribe glucagon to all patients at risk for level 2 or 3 hypoglycemia and instruct caregivers, school personnel, or family members on its use.

Type 2 Diabetes Mellitus

- Diabetes mellitus type 2 is a common endocrine disorder characterized by variable degrees of insulin resistance and deficiency, resulting in hyperglycemia.
- Potential complications of diabetes mellitus include cardiovascular disease, neuropathy, nephropathy, retinopathy, and increased mortality.
- It is often identified through routine screening beginning in middle age, or through targeted screening of adults of any age with overweight or obesity and with risk factors such as metabolic syndrome, polycystic ovary syndrome, a history of gestational diabetes, or other concerning familial, clinical, or demographic characteristics.
- Evaluation:
    - Type 2 diabetes is frequently asymptomatic, but may present with symptoms typical of hyperglycemia such as polyuria, polydipsia, and polyphagia.
    - Perform blood testing to diagnose diabetes.
        - Diagnostic criteria for diabetes is any of:
            - Random plasma glucose ≥ 200 mg/dL (11.1 mmol/L) with symptoms of hyperglycemia (such as polyuria or polydipsia) or hyperglycemic crisis
            - No unequivocal hyperglycemia, but 2 abnormal test results from either 2 separate test samples or the same sample; abnormal test results include:
                - Fasting plasma glucose ≥ 126 mg/dL (7 mmol/L) (no caloric intake for ≥ 8 hours).
                - 2-hour plasma glucose ≥ 200 mg/dL (11.1 mmol/L) during 75-g oral glucose tolerance test.

- HbA1c ≥ 6.5% (HbA1c may not be accurate for diagnosis with pregnancy, hemoglobinopathy, certain anemias, or abnormal erythrocyte loss or replacement).

- Additional testing for diabetic complications:
    - Assess the patient's estimated glomerular filtration rate (calculated from serum creatinine) at least annually.
    - Assess liver transaminases (alanine aminotransferase and aspartate aminotransferase) at the time of diagnosis and annually thereafter to assess for nonalcoholic fatty liver disease.
    - Measure urine albumin, such as urine albumin-to-creatinine ratio, at least annually.
    - Perform a dilated and comprehensive eye examination at the time of diagnosis.
        - If there is no evidence of retinopathy at ≥ 1 annual eye exam in patients with well-controlled glycemia, consider screening every 1-2 years.
        - If any evidence of retinopathy is detected, subsequent dilated retinal exams should be repeated at least annually.
        - More frequent eye exams are required if the retinopathy is progressive or sight-threatening.

- Management:
    - Individualize glycemic goals:
        - HbA1c < 7% (53 mmol/mol) is a reasonable goal for many nonpregnant adults without significant hypoglycemia.
        - More stringent target, such as HbA1c < 6.5% (48 mmol/mol), may be reasonable if it can be achieved without significant hypoglycemia or other adverse effects of

treatment (such as polypharmacy) for selected patients, such as those with:

- Short duration of diabetes.
- Long life expectancy.
- No significant cardiovascular disease.

- Less stringent target, such as HbA1c < 8% (64 mmol/mol), may be appropriate for patients with:

  - History of severe hypoglycemia.
  - Limited life expectancy.
  - Harms of treatment likely to outweigh the benefits.

o Lifestyle modifications:

- Provide support for dietary management, maintaining physical activity, and diabetes self-management education and support.
- This can be done individually (by the clinician, certified diabetes educators, and nurses), in a group setting, or via telemedicine.

Diabetic Ketoacidosis (DKA)

- DKA is an acute complication occurring in patients with diabetes, primarily patients with type 1 diabetes.
- DKA is characterized by both hyperglycemia and anion gap metabolic acidosis.
- Causes:
    - Inadequate insulin treatment, including non-adherence, in patients with known diabetes.
    - New-onset diabetes.
    - Concurrent infection (most commonly pneumonia or UTI).
- Clinical features:
    - Polydipsia, polyuria, nausea, vomiting, weakness, and lethargy.
    - Dehydration, Kussmaul respirations (deep respirations), fruity odor on breath, and mental status changes.
    - Abdominal pain, headache (may indicate cerebral edema).
- Diagnosis:
    - In acutely ill patients, evaluation and management occur concurrently.
    - Initial testing should include:
        - Serum glucose, electrolytes, ketones, and blood gas.
        - Urine dipstick for ketones and urinalysis.
        - CBC with differential.
        - Renal and liver function tests.
        - ECG (ST depression in hypokalemia, or tall and narrow T wave in hyperkalemia).

- Urine or blood culture (if infection suspected).
- Chest X-ray (if pneumonia suspected).

  o Diagnostic findings for DKA are:

  - Serum glucose > 250 mg/dL (13.88 mmol/L).
  - Serum bicarbonate < 18 mEq/L (18 mmol/L).
  - Presence of serum ketones.
  - Blood pH < 7.3

- Differential diagnosis include:

  o Hyperosmolar hyperglycemic crisis.
  o Other causes of anion gap metabolic acidosis in patients without ketonemia or more than mild acidosis.

- Management:

  o The goal of prompt recognition and treatment is to prevent complications, such as renal failure, shock, and death.
  o Initial rehydration is central to management of DKA. Begin fluid resuscitation with 0.9% saline 1-1.5 L/hour (or 15-20 mL/kg/hour) IV during first hour.
  o After initial fluid bolus, assess hydration status and electrolytes especially potassium.

    - If there is severe dehydration, continue the 0.9% saline IV at 1 L/hour.
    - If there is mild dehydration, reduce the infusion rate to 250-500 mL/hour (4-14 mL/kg/hour) and calculate corrected serum sodium.
    - Continue the 0.9% saline IV if the patient is hyponatremic.
    - Change to 0.45% saline IV if there is no hyponatremia.
    - When the serum glucose falls below 200 mg/dL (11.1 mmol/L), change to 5% dextrose with 0.45% saline IV at 150-250 mL/hour.

- For electrolyte replacement:

    - If the level of serum potassium is < 5.2 mmol/L, give replacement potassium after ensuring that there is adequate renal function (urine output 50 mL/hour).
    - If the serum potassium is < 3.3 mmol/L use 20-30 mEq/hour IV and replace potassium prior to starting insulin to avoid cardiac arrhythmias.

- Insulin:

    - Hold insulin if the potassium level is < 3.3 mmol/L until potassium is replete.
    - Regular insulin 0.1 units/kg IV bolus followed by 0.1 units/kg/hour IV as continuous infusion.
    - Target a drop in glucose of 50-75 mg/dL per hour.
    - If serum glucose does not fall by > 10% (or 50-75 mg/dL) in the first hour, give regular insulin 0.14 units/kg IV bolus, then continue the infusion at the previous rate.
    - When serum glucose falls below 200 mg/dL, decrease infusion rate to 0.02-0.05 units/kg/hour IV or give rapid-acting insulin at 0.1 units/kg SC every 2 hours, and monitor glucose every 2-4 hours, maintaining serum glucose at 150-200 mg/dL until DKA resolves.

- Monitor glucose, electrolytes, BUN, creatinine, and venous pH at least every 2-4 hours until stable.

Thyroid Diseases

Hyperthyroidism:

- The most common cause of non-iatrogenic hyperthyroidism is Graves' Disease.
- <u>Graves' Disease</u>: an autoimmune thyroid disorder in which autoantibodies to the TSH receptors on the thyroid gland results in hyper-functioning of the thyroid gland. A prominent finding is also the "stare" due to the ophthalmic involvement.
- <u>Thyroid storm</u>: an acute hypermetabolic state associated with the sudden release of large amounts of thyroid hormone into circulation, leading to autonomic instability and central nervous system dysfunction such as altered mental status, coma, or seizures.
- Clinical features of hyperthyroidism include:

  o Progressive nervousness, palpitations, weight loss, fine resting tremor, dyspnea on exertion, and difficulty concentrating.
  o Physical findings include a rapid pulse rate and elevated BP, with the systolic pressure increased to a greater extent than diastolic pressure, and atrial fibrillation.
  o Symptoms of thyroid storm include fever, confusion, restlessness, and psychotic-like behavior.

- Causes of hyperthyroidism include:

  o Graves' Disease, autonomous thyroid nodule that secretes thyroxine, and iatrogenic.

- Laboratory and imaging evaluation:

- o Elevated free thyroxine level, usually with a corresponding low TSH level.
- o Further testing for autoimmune antibodies and radionucleotide scanning of the thyroid.

    - The detection of serum thyroid-receptor antibodies is a specific diagnostic test for Graves' Disease.

- o Imaging is performed using either an isotope of technetium-99 m (^{99}mTc) or iodine-123 (^{123}I).

    - In patients with Graves' Disease, these will be diffuse hyperactivity with large amounts of uptake.
    - In contrast, thyroiditis demonstrates patchy uptake with overall reduced activity, reflecting the release of existing hormone rather than the overproduction of new thyroxine.

- Management:

    - o Radioactive iodine is the treatment of choice for Graves' disease in adult patients who are not pregnant.

        - It should not be used in children or breast-feeding mothers.

    - o Antithyroid drugs such as Propylthiouracil (PTU), methimazole, and carbimazole.

        - These drugs work by inhibiting the organification of iodine, and PTU also prevents the peripheral conversion of thyroxine (T_4) to triiodothyronine (T_3), its more active form.
        - PTU has a risk of hepatotoxicity. For this reason, methimazole should be considered the 1st-line agent except when the patient is pregnant.
        - PTU is preferred during the 1st trimester of pregnancy.

- Surgery is reserved for patients in whom medications and radioactive iodine ablation are unacceptable treatment modalities, or in whom a large goiter is present that is either compressing nearby structures or is disfiguring.
- For patient presenting thyroid storm, aggressive initial therapy is essential to prevent complications. Treatment should include the administration of high doses of PTU or methimazole and Beta blockers (to control tachycardia and other peripheral symptoms of thyrotoxicosis). Hydrocortisone is given to prevent possible adrenal crisis.

Hypothyroidism:

- Clinical features of hypothyroidism include:

  - Lethargy, weight gain, hair loss, dry skin, slowed mentation or forgetfulness, constipation, intolerance to cold, and a depressed effect.
  - In older patients, hypothyroidism can be confused with Alzheimer's disease.
  - In women, it is often confused with depression.
  - Physical findings include low BP, bradycardia, non-pitting edema, hair thinning or loss.

- Causes of hypothyroidism include:

  - Hashimoto thyroiditis, iatrogenic causes include post-Graves' Disease thyroid ablation and surgical removal of the thyroid gland.

- Laboratory and imaging evaluation:

  - TSH level is elevated in primary hypothyroidism. Free thyroid levels are low.
  - Patients with secondary hypothyroidism have low or undetectable TSH levels.
  - TRH is important in secondary hypothyroidism.

- Management:

    - Thyroid hormone replacement of 1.6 mcg/kg daily is recommended. (Initial dose 25-50 mcg).
    - Titrate the dose of levothyroxine by 12.5 to 25 mcg per day.
    - Evaluation of TSH levels should be performed 4 to 6 weeks after adjustment of medication.

Section 5: Gastroenterology

Gastroesophageal Reflux Disease (GERD)

- GERD is a condition that develops when the reflux of stomach contents into the esophagus causes troublesome symptoms or complications.
- A dysfunctional lower esophageal sphincter allows reflux of large amounts of gastric juice. Delayed gastric emptying can increase the volume and pressure in the reservoir until the valve mechanism is defeated, leading to GERD.
- Clinical features:

    o Heartburn, Regurgitation.
    o Extraesophageal symptoms include hoarseness, sore throat, throat clearing, chronic cough, nausea, asthma, halitosis, chest pain, erosion of dental enamel, pharyngitis, sinusitis, and recurrent otitis media.

- Diagnosis:

    o Diagnose GERD based on clinical features.
    o Evaluate for non-GERD causes of extraesophageal symptoms before attributing such symptoms to GERD.
    o Perform an upper endoscopy in patients with alarm symptoms (dysphagia, bleeding, anemia, weight loss, recurrent vomiting).
    o Perform pH monitoring and consider esophageal manometry.

- Management:

    o Encourage weight loss if overweight or recent weight gain.
    o Prescribe PPI such as omeprazole 20 mg for 4-8 weeks as empiric therapy to relive symptoms and confirm diagnosis.

- Continue PPI as maintenance therapy daily in patients with history of erosive esophagitis.
- In patients not responding to PPI therapy:
  - Increase dosing to PPI BID, re-evaluate to establish diagnosis and rule out other causes.
- Consider antireflux surgery as an alternative option for long-term treatment in patients responsive to but intolerant of PPIs.
- Surgery is not recommended if not responsive to PPI therapy.

- Complications:

  - Esophageal complications:
    - Chest pain, esophagitis, stricture, Barret esophagus, and adenocarcinoma.

  - Extra-esophageal complications (Cough, laryngitis, asthma, and dental erosions).

Irritable Bowel Syndrome (IBS)

- IBS is a GI syndrome characterized by chronic abdominal pain and altered bowel habits in the absence of any organic cause.
- Risk factors include younger patients and women.
- Clinical manifestations of IBS include both GI and extraintestinal complaints. Chronic abdominal pain usually described as a crampy sensation with variable intensity and periodic exacerbations, emotional stress and eating may exacerbate the pain, while defecation often provides some relief. Altered bowel habits ranging from diarrhea and constipation. Other GI symptoms include GERD, dysphagia, intermittent dyspepsia, non-cardiac chest pain, and increased gas production in the form of flatulence. Extraintestinal symptoms include impaired sexual dysfunction, dysmenorrhea, and increased urinary frequency and urgency.
- Diagnostic criteria based on Rome IV criteria as follows:

    o IBS is defined as recurrent abdominal pain, on average, at least one day per week in the last three months, associated with two or more of the following criteria:

    - Related to defecation.
    - Associated with a change in stool frequency.
    - Associated with a change in stool form (appearance).

- The presence of "alarm" or atypical symptoms which are not compatible with IBS are an indication for referral:

    o Rectal bleeding.
    o Nocturnal or progressive abdominal pain.
    o Weight loss.

- Laboratory abnormalities such as anemia, elevated inflammatory markers, or electrolyte disturbance.

- Investigations is based on the type:

  - IBS with predominant constipation:

    - Radiography.
    - Flexible sigmoidoscopy and colonoscopy if a structural lesion is suspected.

  - IBS with diarrhea:

    - Stool cultures to exclude Giardia in patients with possible exposure.
    - Serum Tissue Transglutaminase (tTG-IgA) antibody to screen for Celiac disease.

  - 24-hour stool collection if osmotic or secretory diarrhea or malabsorption is suspected.

- Management include:

  - Lifestyle and dietary modification, education and reassurance in patients with mild to moderate symptoms.
  - Pharmacological therapy is used if there is moderate to severe symptoms, failure of modification therapy, or there is impairment in quality of life.
  - *IBS with constipation:* Laxatives such as Soluble fiber, Polyethylene glycol, Osmotic laxatives such as Lactulose "initial dose is 17 g of powder dissolved in 8 ounces of water once daily and titrate up or down to a maximum dose of 34 g daily", Lubiprostone 8 mcg twice daily, and Linaclotide 290 mcg daily.
  - *IBS with diarrhea:* Antidiarrheal agents such as Loperamide 2 mg 45 minutes before a meal. Bile acid sequestrants such as Colesevelam 1.875 g twice daily.

- *IBS with abdominal pain:* Antispasmodic such as Mebeverine, Dicyclomine 20 mg orally four times daily as needed. Antidepressants such as TCA may be used in patients with persistent abdominal pain despite antispasmodics and those with coexisting depression.

Acute Gastroenteritis

- Acute gastroenteritis, also known as infectious diarrhea, is inflammation of the gastrointestinal tract that involves the stomach and small intestines.
- Etiologies include bacteria, viruses, parasites, toxins, and drugs.
- Viruses are responsible for a significant percentage of cases affecting patients of all ages.

    o Rotavirus is the leading cause of severe childhood gastroenteritis worldwide.

        ▪ Fecal-oral transmission is the main means of spread.

- In adults, norovirus and Campylobacter are common.
- In children, bacteria accounts for about 15% of cases, with the most common types being E.coli, Salmonella, Shigella, and Campylobacter species.
- Clinical features:

    o Viral gastroenteritis ranges from a self-limited watery diarrheal illness (usually < 1 week) associated with symptoms of nausea, vomiting, anorexia, malaise, or fever, to severe dehydration resulting in hospitalization or even death.

- Diagnosis:

    o In most cases that fit the clinical features of viral gastroenteritis, lab tests are not indicated.
    o If bacterial or protozoal infection is suspected, stool studies for occult blood, WBC, microscopy for protozoa, or bacterial culture may be indicated.

- o When needed, stool rotavirus antigen testing has high sensitivity and specificity and is the most commonly used option.
- o A definitive diagnosis is usually not needed as it does not alter management.

- Management:

  - o Supportive care is the mainstay of treatment, with emphasis on rehydration.
  - o No specific antiviral therapy is presently available.
  - o Use of antiemetics, such as ondansetron, may reduce need for IV rehydration.
  - o To avoid spread:

    - Children should be excluded from school or day care for 24 hours from last diarrheal episode.

  - o An oral live attenuated vaccine is available and recommended for all infants starting at age 6 weeks, unless contraindicated.
  - o Vaccination may be associated with a small risk of intussusception.
  - o If bacterial is suspected, macrolides are the preferred agents.

Acute Cholecystitis

- Acute cholecystitis is acute inflammation of the gallbladder, most commonly associated with obstruction of the cystic duct by gallstones or biliary sludge.
- Acalculous cholecystitis is gallbladder inflammation without stones, and is seen primarily in critically ill patients. It requires a high degree of clinical suspicion, is difficult to diagnose, and is associated with a high mortality rate.
- Risk factors include:

    o Female gender, obesity, hormone replacement therapy, hypertriglyceridemia, sickle cell disease, obesity surgery, weight loss, and gallbladder carcinoma.

- Acute cholecystitis may result in secondary infection, emphysematous cholecystitis, gangrenous cholecystitis, gallstone ileus, and gallbladder perforation (with peritonitis).
- Clinical Features and Diagnosis:

    o Suspect acute cholecystitis if signs of both local inflammation (Murphy sign or right upper quadrant mass, pain, or tenderness) and systemic inflammation (fever, elevated WBC, or elevated C-reactive protein) are present.

    o Consider CT for atypical presentations to assess a wider differential diagnosis.

    o Obtain blood tests to assess severity or comorbidities including a CBC, C-reactive protein, BUN, creatinine, electrolytes, bilirubin, ALT, AST, ALP, and amylase.

    o Classify severity as mild (most cases), moderate if signs of severe inflammation, or severe if there is organ dysfunction.

    o Consider bile cultures in moderate or severe acute cholecystitis.

- Management:

    o Initial management includes providing nothing by mouth, IV fluids, electrolyte correction, and analgesics.
    o For severe or health care-associated acute cholecystitis, give broad-spectrum antibiotics such as metronidazole + a beta-lactam (ciprofloxacin, levofloxacin, or ceftazidime or cefepime); or monotherapy with meropenem, imipenem-clistatin, dorpenem, or piperacillin-tazobactam. Add vancomycin if Enterococcus or health care associated.
    o Perform cholecystectomy within 72 hours in mild acute cholecystitis.
    o Consider delaying cholecystectomy by 4 weeks and performing gallbladder drainage early if there is severe local inflammation and urgently if there is organ dysfunction.

Acute Pancreatitis

- It is an inflammatory condition of the pancreas, characterized by acute epigastric or left upper quadrant abdominal pain that sometimes extends to the back, and worsen in the supine position, associated with nausea and vomiting.
- The most common cause of acute pancreatitis is gallstones causing obstruction of the normal flow of pancreatic fluid and leading to pancreatic injury.
- Other possible causes could be due to high triglyceride levels in the blood, high calcium levels in the blood, or heavy alcohol consumption.
- Diagnosis is confirmed by history, physical examination, and typically a blood test (amylase or lipase levels are elevated 3 times).
- Transabdominal ultrasound is commonly done to evaluate the gallbladder for stones.
- Magnetic Resonance Cholangiopancreatography (MRCP) and CT scan is done to confirm the diagnosis if there is uncertainty.
- Severity can be assessed by:

  o Revised Atlanta Criteria:

    - *Mild acute pancreatitis:* absence of extrapancreatic organ failure, local or systemic complications.
    - *Moderate acute pancreatitis:* presence of complications such as peripancreatic fluid collection or necrosis, systemic complications without persistent organ failure.
    - *Severe acute pancreatitis:* presence of organ failure that persists after 48 hours.

- Ranson's Criteria:

    - Age > 55 years.
    - WBCs count > 16,000 cells/mm3.
    - Blood glucose > 200 mg/dL.
    - Serum AST > 250 IU/L.
    - Serum LDH > 350 IU/L.

    If the score is 3 or higher, severe pancreatitis is likely.
    If the score is less than 3, severe pancreatitis is unlikely.

- Management is done by admitting the patient to an ICU if there is organ failure, provide aggressive hydration (such as Lactated Ringer's 250-500 mL/hour) and reassess fluid requirements at frequent intervals within 6 hours of admission for the next 48 hours to achieve decrease in blood urea nitrogen, provide analgesia, provide enteral nutrition instead of parenteral nutrition, prescribe antibiotics for extrapancreatic infection, perform Endoscopic Retrograde Cholangiopancreatography (ERCP) within 24 hours for patients with gallstone pancreatitis with cholangitis, and don't perform drainage or debridement for asymptomatic pancreatic pseudocysts or necrosis "regardless of size or location".
- If infected necrosis is suspected, obtain a CT-guided fine-needle aspiration for Gram stain and culture to guide antibiotic selection, or provide empiric antibiotics with one of the following:

    - Imipenem-Cilastain 500 mg IV every 8 hours.
    - Meropenem 1 g IV every 8 hours.
    - Ciprofloxacin 400 mg IV every 12 hours plus Metronidazole 500 mg IV every 8 hours.

- In patients with gallstones, perform cholecystectomy before discharge if mild, or after active inflammation and fluid collections resolve or stabilize if severe.
- To decrease risk of recurrence, treat alcohol abuse and triglyceride levels.

Charcot's Triad
Fever + RUQ Pain + Jaundice

Reynold's Pentad
Charcot's Triad + AMS + Hypotension

Peptic Ulcer Disease (PUD)

- PUD is a mucosal defect in the gastric or duodenal wall that extends through muscularis mucosa (innermost layer of mucosa) into deeper layers of wall (submucosa or muscularis propria).
- Most peptic ulcers are caused by H. Pylori or NSAIDs, including aspirin.
- Bleeding is the most common frequent and severe complication of PUD. Other complications include perforation and gastric outlet obstruction.
- For patients on chronic NSAIDs, consider primary ulcer prophylaxis with PPI if there are multiple risk factors for PUD, such as age > 60 years and concomitant use of aspirin, anticoagulants, or corticosteroids.
- Evaluation:

  - Patients may present with episodic, gnawing epigastric pain which may be relieved by eating, antacids, or antisecretory agents and can occur with fasting or at night.
  - PUD is usually diagnosed based on endoscopy:

    - Perform upper endoscopy if there are alarm symptoms such as unintentional weight loss, abdominal mass, melena, or hemodynamic instability.
    - Consider endoscopy in patients > 55 years old with unexplained persistent dyspepsia.
    - For patients with uncomplicated dyspepsia (when endoscopy is not indicated), a test-and-treat strategy for H. Pylori is recommended.

  - If not already done, test for H. Pylori in any patient with PUD.
  - Consider biopsy for most gastric ulcers seen on endoscopy, but do not routinely biopsy duodenal ulcers due to low likelihood of malignancy.

- Management:

    o For ulcers while taking NSAIDs-stop NSAIDs if possible, provide PPI or histamine-2 receptor (H2) blocker for 8 weeks, and subsequently add H. Pylori eradication if H. Pylori positive.
    o For H. Pylori-positive ulcers:

        ▪ Provide H. Pylori eradication therapy. A common regimen of choice is 10-14 days of 3 drugs twice daily: a PPI, clarithromycin 500 mg, and either amoxicillin 1 g or metronidazole 500 mg.
        ▪ Following H. Pylori eradication therapy, consider an additional 3 weeks of PPI for patients with gastric ulcers, but additional acid suppression therapy appears unnecessary after successful H. Pylori eradication for duodenal ulcers.
        ▪ For H. Pylori-positive ulcers, consider retesting with C-13 urea breath test (or stool antigen test if urea breath test unavailable) ≥ 4 weeks after treatment to confirm H. Pylori eradication, especially if unresponsive to therapy. For gastric ulcers, consider repeating endoscopy at 6-8 weeks to confirm healing.

    o Treat H. Pylori-negative ulcers in patients not using NSAIDs with PPI or H2 blocker for 4-8 weeks.
    o For patients continuing to take NSAIDs following ulcer healing, offer gastric protection with PPI or substitute a cyclooxygenase-2 (COX-2) NSAID, but also provide ongoing assessment of need for NSAID. Consider that COX-2 NSAIDs may increase risk for cardiovascular events.
    o For symptom recurrence in patients with negative evaluation for malignancy or persistent H. Pylori infection, consider maintenance antisecretory therapy with PPI at lowest dose or with an "as needed approach".
    o Surgery is indicated for perforated peptic ulcers. Consider surgery in selected patients unable to be treated medically.

Diverticulitis

- Diverticulitis refers to inflamed diverticula, which are abnormal but common outpunching of the GI lumen. It happens due to weakened colonic muscle wall resistance.
- Risk factors for the development and/or progression of diverticulosis include increasing age, constipation, low dietary fiber intake, obesity, lack of exercise, and NSAIDs use.
- The consumption of nuts, corn or popcorn, and berries has not been associated with an increased risk for the development of diverticulitis or bleeding from diverticula.
- Clinical features include:

  o Acute diverticulitis typically presents in older adults with acute onset of constant abdominal pain (usually left lower quadrant), often with fever and leukocytosis.
  o Other possible symptoms include

    - Constipation, nausea, vomiting, diarrhea, dysuria, anorexia.

  o Signs of peritonitis, hypotension, or tachycardia often indicate complicated diverticulitis.
  o Symptoms of complicated diverticulitis include:

    - Severe abdominal pain increasing with movement.
    - Palpitations/racing heartbeat.
    - Symptoms specific to organs involved with fistulizing diverticulitis:

      - Colovesical fistulas: pneumaturia, fecaluria, pyria.
      - Colovaginal fistulas: stool passing through vagina.
      - Enterocolonic fistulas: severe diarrhea.

- Rebound tenderness, rigidity, and absence of bowel sounds may suggest peritonitis.
- Rectal exam may reveal tenderness or mass, especially with low-lying pelvic abscess.
- DDx include: appendicitis, IBS, IBD, colon cancer, UTI, or gynecological disorders.

- Diagnosis:

  - A clinical diagnosis of acute diverticulitis can often be made based on history and physical findings, especially in patients with known diverticulosis of previously confirmed diverticulitis.
  - In addition to history and physical exam, the initial evaluation of acute diverticulitis should include a CBC, urinalysis to rule out a UTI, and in selected cases, a plain abdominal X-ray looking for free air under the diaphragm indicative of macroperforation.
  - CT of the abdomen and pelvis is usually the most appropriate imaging modality.
  - Colonoscopy is generally contraindicated in cases of acute diverticulitis but may be useful 4-6 weeks after symptoms resolve in cases of complicated diverticulitis to rule out malignancy.

- Management:

  - Consider outpatient management for patients with mild symptoms. Otherwise hospitalize patients with diverticulitis.
  - Diet:
    - In outpatients, advice clear liquid diet for 2-3 days.
    - In outpatients, NPO until symptoms improve.
  - If antibiotic use is deemed appropriate, suggested oral regimens for mild uncomplicated diverticulitis include:

- Trimethoprim-Sulfamethoxazole DS 160/800 mg orally every 12 hours.
- Ciprofloxacin 750 mg orally every 12 hours plus metronidazole 500 mg orally every 6 hours.
- Levofloxacin 750 mg PO once daily plus metronidazole 500 mg PO every 6 hours.

o Antibiotic choices for inpatients with mild-moderate symptoms include:

- Piperacillin-tazobactam 3.375 g IV every 6 hours or 4.5 g IV every 8 hours.
- Ticarcillin-clavulanate 3.1 g IV every 6 hours.
- Ertapenem 1 g IV every 24 hours.
- Moxifloxacin 400 mg IV every 24 hours.

o For inpatients with severe symptoms, use any of the following as first-line options:

- Imipenem-cilastatin 500 mg IV every 6 hours.
- Meropenem 1 g IV every 8 hours.
- Doripenem 500 mg IV every 8 hours.

o Uncomplicated diverticulitis should improve within 2-4 days of antibiotic treatment with inpatient or outpatient management. In the absence of improvement with medical management. Suspect complicated diverticulitis and perform additional imaging.

- Complicated diverticulitis refers to inflammation of colonic diverticula associated with perforation, bleeding, obstruction, fistula, phlegmon, or abscess.

- Consider adding rifaximin, mesalazine, and/or probiotics in patients with persistent symptoms after resolution of acute diverticulitis.
- Surgery may be considered if symptoms do not improve with medical management, or there is evidence of phlegm, fistula, obstruction, or in multiquadrant peritonitis.
- Surgical options include laparoscopic or open approaches for drainage, washout, or resection (e.g., hemicolectomy).

Hepatic Encephalopathy

- Hepatic encephalopathy is defined as a spectrum of neuropsychiatric abnormalities in patients with liver dysfunction, after exclusion of brain disease.
- It is characterized by personality changes, intellectual impairment, and a depressed level of consciousness.
- Pathophysiology:

    o Astrocytes account for about one third of the cortical volume. The play a key role in the regulation of the blood-brain barrier. They are involved in maintaining electrolyte homeostasis and in providing nutrients and neurotransmitter precursors to neurons. They also play a role in the detoxification of a number of chemicals, including ammonia. It is theorized that neurotoxic substances, including ammonia and manganese, may gain entry into the brain in the setting of liver failure. These neurotoxic substances may then contribute to morphologic changes in astrocytes.

- Clinical features include:

    o Grading of the symptoms of hepatic encephalopathy is performed according to the so-called West Haven classification system, as follows:

        ▪ *Grade 0*: minimal hepatic encephalopathy (also known as Covert Hepatic Encephalopathy "CHE" and previously known subclinical hepatic encephalopathy); lack of detectable changes in personality or behavior; minimal changes in memory, concentration, intellectual function, and coordination; asterixis is absent.

- - - *Grade 1*: trivial lack of awareness; shortened attention span; impaired addition or subtraction; hypersomnia, insomnia, or inversion of sleep pattern; euphoria, depression, or irritability; mild confusion; slowing of ability to perform mental tasks.
    - *Grade 2*: lethargy of apathy; disorientation; inappropriate behavior; slurred speech; obvious asterixis; drowsiness; gross deficits in ability to perform mental tasks, obvious personality changes, inappropriate behavior, and intermittent disorientation, usually regarding time.
    - *Grade 3*: somnolent but can be aroused; unable to perform mental tasks; disorientation about time and place; marked confusion; amnesia; occasional fits of rage; present but incomprehensible speech.
    - *Grade 4*: coma with or without response to painful stimuli.
  - Grades 0 and 1 are said CHE, grades 2 through 4 are said overt hepatic encephalopathy (OHE).

- Common precipitants of hepatic encephalopathy include:

  - *Renal failure*: leads to decreased clearance of urea, ammonia.
  - *GI bleeding*: results in increased ammonia and nitrogen absorption from gut. Bleeding may predispose to kidney hypoperfusion and impaired renal function.
  - *Constipation*: increases intestinal production and absorption of ammonia.
  - *Medications*: drug that act upon the CNS, such as opiates, benzodiazepines, antidepressants, and antipsychotic agents, may worsen hepatic encephalopathy.

- Differential Diagnosis:

  - *Intracranial lesions*, such as subdural hematoma, intracranial bleeding, stroke, tumor, abscess.
  - *Infections*, such as meningitis, encephalitis, and intracranial abscess.

- *Metabolic encephalopathy*, such as hypoglycemia, electrolyte imbalance, anoxia, hypercarbia.
- Hyperammonemia from other causes, such as ureterosigmoidostomy.

- Diagnosis:

  - Suspect HE in patients with liver cirrhosis who have changes in mental status, or behaviors.
  - Patients may have signs of liver diseases such as jaundice, ascites, spider angiomata, and flapping asterixis.
  - Diagnostic workup required to rule out other disorders that can alter brain function.
  - Elevated blood ammonia level is the classic lab abnormality reported in patients with HE.
  - CT and MRI of the brain may be important in ruling out intracranial lesion.

- Management:

  - Identify and correct precipitating factors and alternative causes of altered mental status.
  - Maintain nutrition with protein intake of 1.2-1.5 g/kg/day and energy intake of 35-40 kcal/kg of ideal body weight.
  - Use lactulose (45 mL orally every hour acutely until defecation, then 15-45 mL every 8-12 hours to maintain 2-3 stools per day) for treatment of episodic OHE and then continue for prevention of recurrent episodes.
  - Use Rifaximin 550 mg orally twice daily as add-on to lactulose for the prevention of recurrent episodes after second episode of hepatic encephalopathy

Section 6: Geriatric

Delirium

- Delirium is a common complication in the hospital setting.
- Delirium may be differentiated from dementia by its acute onset and waxing and waning mental state.
- Elderly patients, especially those with a history of dementia, and the severely ill are at greatest risk of developing delirium.
- Delirium may be precipitated by medications, post-surgical state, infection, or electrolyte imbalance.
- The management of delirium relies on non-pharmacologic approaches, including:

    o Frequent reorientation.
    o Discontinuation of any unnecessary noxious stimuli (e.g., urinary catheters, unnecessary oxygen delivery systems or telemetry monitors, and restraints).

    - Physical or chemical restraints actually impair recovery from delirium and should be used only as a last resort to prevent serious harm to self or others.

    o Environmental modification to establish day/night sleep cycles.
    o Discontinuation of unnecessary medications.

    - Benzodiazepines frequently induce a delirium and their continued use or escalation may impair recovery.
    - Fluoroquinolones can worsen mental status in the elderly.

Dementia

- Dementia is a clinical syndrome marked by an acquired impairment of memory, cognition, or language abilities, sufficient to impair functioning.
- Dementia is a meaningful decline from previous level of cognitive performance in ≥ 1 cognitive domains (complex attention, executive function, learning and memory, language, perceptual-motor, or social cognition) and the cognitive deficits interfere with independence in everyday activities.
- Rapidly progressive dementia is dementia developing within 24 months after appearance of first cognitive symptoms.
- Early-onset dementia is dementia in patient < 65 years old.
- Mild cognitive impairment (MCI) is impairment of memory or other cognitive functions which has slight or no effect on patient's functional abilities.
- Delirium is fluctuating, acute confusional state with disturbance in consciousness and change in cognition.
- Common causes of irreversible dementia include neurodegenerative dementing illnesses (such as Alzheimer disease, dementia with Lewy bodies, and frontotemporal dementia) and vascular dementia.
- Potential reversible causes of impaired cognitive function include depression, delirium, seizure, infections, inflammatory brain diseases, metabolic abnormalities, brain lesions, and medication exposures.
- Evaluation:

  o Suspect dementia in patients with a decline in functioning and an impaired ability to function at work or at usual activities as reported by the patient or a reliable informant.
  o Conduct a history and physical exam to identify potentially reversible causes and to assess the functional status of the patient.

- When possible, obtain corroborative information form a collateral source who knows the patient well and can interpret current symptoms relative to past performance.
- Assess and document the level of consciousness, orientation, cognition, attention, speech and language, and recent and remote memory.
- Assess activities of daily living.

o Obtain blood tests including CBC, electrolytes, glucose, calcium, RFT, LFT, TSH, vitamin B12, folate, and ESR to evaluate for reversible causes of dementia.
o Perform a "bedside" cognitive assessment using 1 of the various standardized tests, such as the Mini-Mental State Examination.
o Perform cerebral imaging (CT or MRI) for all patients with evidence of cognition impairment or dementia.
o EEG should not be used as a routine investigation in persons with dementia. Consider EEG in assessment of associated seizure disorder in patient with dementia.
o Assess for decision-making competency to determine the level of support needed.
o Encourage patients to draft advance directives specifying their wishes for future treatment and care preferences.
o Consider identifying patients at an increased risk for unsafe driving.

Section 7: Hematology

Classification of Anemia

- Anemia is defined as:

    o Hemoglobin (Hb) level < 12 g/dL (120 g/L) in non-pregnant women > 15 years old.
    o Hb level < 14 g/dL in males > 15 years.
    o Hb level < 12.5 g/dL in children aged 5-11 years (adults).
    o Hb level < 11 g/dL in pregnant women, or children aged 6-59 months.

Sickle Cell Anemia

- Sickle cell disease (SCD) refers to any one of the syndromes in which the sickle mutation is co-inherited with a mutation at the other beta globin allele that reduces or abolishes normal beta globin production. These include sickle cell anemia (SCA), sickle beta thalassemia, hemoglobin SC disease, and others.
- SCD is a group of chronic hemolytic anemias with autosomal recessive inheritance caused by presence of ≥ 1 sickle hemoglobin gene, leading to $> 50\%$ production of hemoglobin S (HbS). HbS polymerizes when deoxygenated, distorting RBCs and causing a characteristic sickle shape.
- Sickle cell trait is a benign carrier condition, usually with none of the symptoms of SCA or other SCDs.

    o If both parents have the sickle cell trait, the chance that a child will have sickle cell disease is 25%.
    o If one parent is carrying the trait and the other actually has disease, the odds increase to 50% that their child will inherit the disease.

- SCA is a disease of RBCs caused by an autosomal-recessive single gene defect in the beta chain of hemoglobin (HbA), which results in sickle cell hemoglobin (HbS).
- Causes:

    o The sickling process that prompts a crisis (i.e., vaso-occlusive crises) may be precipitated by multiple factors:

        ▪ Local tissue hypoxia, dehydration secondary to a viral illness, or nausea and vomiting, all of which lead to hypertonicity of the plasma, may induce sickling.
        ▪ Any event that can lead to acidosis, such as infection or extreme dehydration, can cause sickling.

- More benign factors and environmental changes, such as fatigue, exposure to cold, and psychosocial stress, can elicit the sickling process.

  o Vaso-occlusive crisis occurs when the microcirculation is obstructed by sickled RBCs, causing ischemic injury to the organ supplied and resultant pain.

- Clinical features include:

  o The most common clinical manifestation of SCA is vaso-occlusive crisis.
  o Pain crises constitute the most distinguishing clinical feature of SCD and are the leading cause of ED visits and hospitalizations for affected patients.
  o Pain crises begin suddenly. The crisis may last several hours to several days and terminates as abruptly as it began.
  o The pain can affect any body part. It often involves the abdomen, bones, joints, and soft tissue, and it may present as dactylitis (bilateral painful and swollen hands and/or feet in children).
  o Aplastic crisis:

    - It is a serious complication, caused by infection with Parvovirus B-19. A normally benign childhood disorder associated with fever, malaise, and a mild rash.
    - The virus infects RBC progenitor in the bone marrow, resulting in impaired cell division for a few days. The condition is self-limited, with bone marrow recovery occurring in 7-10 days, followed by brisk reticulocytosis.

  o Splenic sequestration:

    - It occurs with highest frequency during the first 5 years of life in children with SCA.
    - It can occur at any age in individuals with other sickle syndromes.

- This complication is characterized by the onset of life-threatening anemia with rapid enlargement of the spleen and high reticulocyte count.
- It is a medical emergency that demands prompt and appropriate treatment.

o Infants with SCD may develop hand-foot syndrome.

- It is not seen after 5 years because hematopoiesis in the small bones of the hands and feet ceases at this age.

o Acute chest syndrome:

- In young children, the acute chest syndrome consists of chest pain, fever, cough, tachypnea, leukocytosis, and pulmonary infiltrates in the upper lobes.
- Adults are usually afebrile and dyspneic with severe chest pain and multilobar and lower lobe disease.
- It is a medical emergency and should be treated immediately, to prevent ARDS.

o CNS involvement is one of the most devastating aspects of SCD.

- It is most prevalent in childhood and adolescence. The most severe manifestation is stroke (affecting 30% of children and 11% of patients by 20 years).
- It is usually ischemic in children and hemorrhagic in adults.
- Hemiparesis is the usual presentation.

o Cardiac involvement:

- The heart is involved due to chronic anemia and microinfarcts. Hemolysis and blood transfusion lead to hemosiderin deposition in the myocardium.

- Physical findings are not specific (e.g., scleral icterus, splenomegaly). It is important to perform a neurological exam and look for underlying cause based on the clinical presentation.

- Diagnosis:

    - Typical baseline abnormalities in the patient with SCD are as follows:

        - Hemoglobin level is 5-9 g/dL.
        - Hematocrit is decreased to 17-29%.
        - Leukocytosis with a predominance of neutrophils.
        - Platelet count is increased.
        - ESR is low.
        - The reticulocyte count is usually elevated.
        - Peripheral blood smears demonstrate target cells, elongated cells, and characteristic sickle erythrocytes.
        - Presence of RBCs containing nuclear remnants (Howell-Jolly bodies) indicates that the patient is asplenic.

    - Sickling test will establish the presence of HbS gene.
    - Chest radiography should be performed in patients with respiratory symptoms.
    - MRI can demonstrate avascular necrosis of the femoral and humeral heads and may distinguish between osteomyelitis and bony infarction in patients with bone pain.
    - Transcranial Doppler Ultrasonography (TCD) can identify children with SCD who are at high risk stroke by documenting abnormality high blood flow velocity in the large arteries of the circle of Willis (the middle cerebral or internal carotid arteries).
    - In patients with abdominal pain, abdominal US can be used to rule out cholecystitis, cholelithiasis, or an ectopic pregnancy and to measure spleen and liver size.

- Management:

    o Patient education:
        - Patients must be educated about the nature of their disease. They must be able to recognize the earliest signs of a vaso-occlusive crisis and seek help, treat all febrile illness promptly, and identify environmental hazards that may precipitate a crisis.

    o The goals of management include fluid replacement therapy, pain management, and symptom control.
    o Fluid therapy:

        - Normal saline and 5% dextrose is saline may be used.

    o Pain management:

        - Pain management should include 4 stages: (assessment, treatment, reassessment, and adjustment).
        - For severe pain, rapidly initiate parenteral opioids.
        - Chronic pain is managed with long-acting oral morphine preparations and acetaminophen and NSAIDs.
        - Opioids analgesics:

            ❖ <u>Codeine</u>: is used to treat mild to moderate pain.
            ❖ <u>Oxycodone</u>: is indicated for the relief of moderate to severe pain.
            ❖ <u>Morphine sulfate</u>: is used to treat moderate to severe pain.
            ❖ <u>Methadone</u>: is used in the treatment of severe pain.
            ❖ <u>Fentanyl</u>: is 50-100 times more potent than morphine.

        - NSAIDs include:

            ❖ Aspirin.
            ❖ Acetaminophen.
            ❖ Ibuprofen.

- Control of symptoms:

    - In patients with acute chest syndrome, supplemental oxygen is recommended.
    - Use antimetabolites (e.g., hydroxyurea) for adults with SCA with ≥ 3 crises with moderate-to-severe pain in a 12-month period or in those with sickle cell interferes with daily activities and quality of life.
    - Transfusions are not needed for the usual anemia or episodes of pain associated with SCD. Urgent replacement of blood is often required for sudden, severe anemia due to acute splenic sequestration, parvovirus B19 infection, or hyperhemolytic crises. With continued transfusion, iron overload inevitably develops and can result in heart and liver failure and multiple other complications. Three agents are available for iron chelation: Desferrioxamine, Deferasirox, and Deferiprone.
    - Folic acid is necessary for proper nucleotide metabolism. It is an important cofactor for enzymes used in the production of RBCs.

Multiple Myeloma

- Multiple myeloma (MM) is characterized by a proliferation of malignant plasma cells and a subsequent overabundance of monoclonal paraprotein (M protein).

    o Malignant clonal bone marrow plasma cell tumor with excessive M protein production.

- It is a debilitating malignancy that is part of a spectrum of diseases ranging from monoclonal gammopathy of unknown significance (MGUS) to plasma cell leukemia.
- The new definition of active multiple myeloma is:

    o Clonal bone marrow plasma cells ≥ 10% or biopsy-proven bony or extramedullary plasmacytoma and any one or more of the following CRAB features and myeloma-defining events:

    - *Hypercalcemia*: serum calcium > 0.25 mmol/L (1 mg/dL) higher than the upper limit of normal > 2.75 mmol/L (11 mg/dL).
    - *Renal insufficiency*: creatinine clearance < 40 mL per minute or serum creatinine > 177 μmol/L (> 2 mg/dL).
    - *Anemia*: hemoglobin value of > 29 g/L below the lowest limit of normal, or a hemoglobin value of < 100 g/L.
    - *Bone lesions*: one or more osteolytic lesion on skeletal radiography, CT, or PET/CT. if bone marrow has < 10% clonal plasma cells, more than one bone lesion is required to distinguish from solitary plasmacytoma with minimal marrow involvement.

- o Any one or more of the following biomarkers of malignancy (MDEs):

    - 60% or greater clonal plasma cells on bone marrow examination.
    - Serum involved / uninvolved free light chain ratio of 100 or greater, provided the absolute level of the involved light chain is at least 100 mg/L.
    - More than one focal lesion on MRI that is at least 5 mm or greater in size.
    - Classification (based on International Myeloma Working Group):

- o MGUS:

    - Serum M protein < 30 g/L.
    - Clonal bone marrow plasma cells < 10%.
    - Absence of end-organ damage such as hypercalcemia, renal insufficiency, anemia, and bone lesions (CRAB) or amyloidosis that can be attributed to the plasma cell proliferative disorder.

- o Asymptomatic myeloma (smoldering myeloma):

    - Serum M protein > 30 g/L.
    - Bone marrow clonal plasma cells > 10%.
    - No related organ damage.

- o Symptomatic MM:

    - Serum and/or urine M protein.
    - Bone marrow (clonal) plasma cells or plasmacytoma.
    - Related end-organ impairment.

- o Non-secretory myeloma:

- No M protein in serum and/or urine with immunofixation.
- Bone marrow clonal plasmacytosis > 10% or plasmacytoma.
- Related end-organ damage.

- Solitary plasmacytoma of bone:
    - No M protein and/or urine.
    - Single area of bone destruction due to clonal plasma cells (multiple solitary plasmacytomas if > 1 localized area of bone destruction or extramedullary tumor of clonal plasma cells which may be recurrent).
    - Bone marrow not consistent with MM.
    - No related organ or tissue impairment.

- Extramedullary plasmacytoma:

    - No M protein in serum and/or urine.
    - Extramedullary tumor of clonal plasma cells.
    - Normal bone marrow.
    - Normal skeletal survey.
    - No related end-organ damage.
    - Clinical features:

- The presentation of MM can range from asymptomatic to severely symptomatic, with complications requiring emergent treatment.
- Systemic ailments include bleeding, infection, and renal failure; pathologic fractures and spinal cord compression may occur.
- Presenting symptoms of MM include the following:

    - Bone pain.
    - Weakness, malaise.
    - Bleeding, anemia.
    - Infection (often pneumococcal).
    - Hypercalcemia.
    - Neuropathies.

- Diagnosis:

    o MM is often discovered through routine blood screening when patients are being evaluated for unrelated problems.
    o In one third of patients, the condition is diagnosed after a pathologic fracture occurs, usually involving the axial skeleton.

- Investigations:

    o The international Myeloma Workshop guidelines for standard investigative work-up in patients with suspected MM includes the following:

        - Serum and urine assessment for monoclonal protein (densitometer tracing and nephelometric quantitation; immunofixation for confirmation).
        - Serum free light chain assay (in all patients with newly diagnosed plasma cell dyscrasisas).
        - Bone marrow aspiration and/or biopsy.
        - Serum beta2-microglobulin, albumin, and lactate dehydrogenase measurement.
        - Standard metaphase cytogenetics.
        - Fluorescence in situ hybridization.
        - Skeletal survey.
        - MRI for detecting thoracic and lumbar spine lesions, paraspinal involvement, and early cord compression.

- Management:

    o There is currently no cure for MM. However, advances in therapy, such as autologous stem cell transplantation, radiation, and surgical care in certain cases, have helped to lessen the occurrence and severity of adverse effects of this disease and to manage associated complications.
    o Chemotherapy regimens used in patients with MM include the following:

- Thalidomide, either as single agent or in combination with steroids or melphalan.
- Lenalidomide plus dexamethasone.
- Bortezomib plus melphalan.
- VAD (vincristine, doxorubicin "Adriamycin", and dexamethasone).
- Melphalan plus prednisone.

o Adding bisphosphonates to treatment of myeloma may reduce pathological vertebral fractures and pain but may not reduce mortality.
o Treat any febrile myeloma patient promptly with broad-spectrum antibiotics, avoiding aminoglycosides if possible.

Henoch-Schoenlein Purpura

- HSP also known as anaphylactoid purpura, is a generalized, acute systemic immune-mediated small vasculitis of unknown cause involving small blood vessels.
- Clinical features:

  o Skin lesion (palpable purpura, erythematous maculopapular and petechial lesions).
  o Colicky abdominal pain.
  o Vomiting.
  o Melena.
  o Renal involvement (hematuria and proteinuria).
  o Arthritis or arthralgia.

- Diagnosis:

  o Diagnosis of HSP is often clinical.
  o The platelet count, serum complement, and IgA levels (which may be demonstrated on skin or kidney biopsy) can be normal or elevated.
  o Coagulation studies are normal.

- Management:

  o HSP is usually self-limited and lasts about 4 weeks, although the recurrence rate is high up to 40%.
  o Treatment often only requires supportive care with attention to hydration and nutrition.
  o For external manifestations (such as joint pain or abdominal pain), consider acetaminophen and corticosteroids.

- o Monitoring for development of HSP nephritis (HSPN) is suggested for 12 months following diagnosis.

    - If there is persistent proteinuria $> 0.5\text{-}1$ g/day/1.73 mm^2, consider ACEI or ARB.

- o Don't use corticosteroids to prevent HSPN.

- Complications:

    - o Renal complications and long-term renal involvement are common in adults.

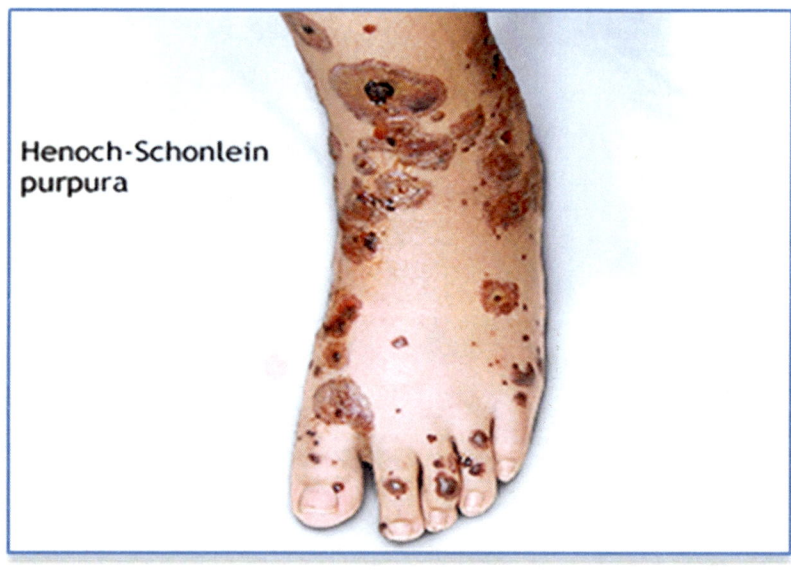

Henoch-Schonlein purpura

Idiopathic Thrombocytopenic Purpura

- ITP is an acquired autoimmune disorder characterized by the immune-mediated destruction of otherwise normal platelet.
- ITP is defined by a platelet count < 100×10^9 /L in the absence of other causes of thrombocytopenia.
- Classification:

  o Primary ITP:
  - Arises without an obvious initiating or underlying cause.

  o Secondary ITP:
  - It is due to an underlying disease (SLE, HIV, HCV) or drug exposure (Quinine, Penicillin).

- Clinical features:

  o Most patients are asymptomatic or present with an abrupt onset of mucocutaneous bleeding.
  o Most common manifestation of bleeding is purpura, particularly petechiae and ecchymoses on the extensor surfaces of the skin, and easily bruises.
  o A viral illness may precede the onset of thrombocytopenia.

- Diagnosis:

  o ITP is a diagnosis of exclusion.
  o Baseline tests include a CBC and a peripheral blood smear.
  o Consider testing for acute and chronic viral infections (e.g., B19, HCV).

- o A bone marrow examination is not required in children and adolescents who present with typical features of ITP.

- Management:

  - o In children with acute ITP and mild-clinical disease, watchful waiting is considered the first-line therapy; monitor with supportive advice.
  - o For the treatment of children with moderate bleeding or increased risk of bleeding, administer 1 of the following:

    - Prednisone 1-2 mg/kg/day for a maximum of 14 days, titrated to platelet count with rapid tapering.
    - IVIG single dose 0.8-1 g/kg, especially if a more rapid increase in platelet count is desired or as an alternative to steroid therapy.

  - o Splenectomy is rarely indicated, but consider it in children and adolescents with persistent or significant bleeding, and intolerance or lack of response to less invasive, 1st-line therapies.

Section 8: Infectious Diseases

Viral Hepatitis

- Hepatitis is an inflammation of the liver that is characterized by nausea, anorexia, fever, right-upper abdominal discomfort, jaundice, and marked elevation of LFTs.

- *Hepatitis A:*

    o Also known as infectious hepatitis, the causative agent is an RNA virus.
    o The onset of clinical symptoms is usually acute, and children and young adults are usually affected.
    o The transmission is via a fecal-oral route and has been linked to the consumption of contaminated shellfish (e.g., raw oysters).
    o The course of the disease is usually mild, and the prognosis is usually excellent.
    o There is neither an associated chronic state nor a carrier state.
    o The diagnosis is made by the detection of elevated levels of IgM antibodies, which indicate active disease, and IgG antibodies, which indicate previous disease.
    o Most cases require no special treatment other than supportive care, and symptoms usually resolve after several weeks.
    o The disease can be prevented by administering Ig to those who are in close contact with those affected. Immunization, especially for travelers, is recommended to specifically prevent hepatitis A.

- *Hepatitis B:*

    o This DNA viral disease is more severe than hepatitis A and causes more complications.
    o The disease often develops insidiously and can affect persons of all ages.

- It is transmitted parenterally (through infected blood transfusions or infected needles used by IV drug abusers) and through sexual contact (especially in sexually active young adults and homosexuals).
- Approximately 10% of cases become chronic; up to 30% of affected patients become carriers of the virus after they are infected.
- The detection of the hepatitis B surface antigen supports the diagnosis of acute illness, and values become positive between 1 and 7 weeks before the symptoms become evident.
- The hepatitis B antibody appears weeks to months after the development of the clinical symptoms.
- The presence of a hepatitis B surface antibody indicates previous disease and represents immunity.
- Those who have received hepatitis B vaccination also have positive titers if they are immune.
- An anticore antibody (IgM) usually develops at the onset of the illness, and the IgG anticore antibody (which develops shortly after IgM appears) can be used as a marker for the disease during the "window period", which occurs when the hepatitis B surface antigen disappears and before the hepatitis B surface antibodies appear.
- The presence of hepatitis B e antigen is associated with greater infectivity and a greater chance of progression to the chronic state.
- Prophylaxis of hepatitis B can be achieved with hepatitis B vaccine given at 1 month and 6 months after the initial injection, for a total of 3 injections.
- Persons exposed to hepatitis B (e.g., by needle stick) should also receive hepatitis B Ig at time of exposure.

- *Hepatitis C:*

    - It is transmitted by infected blood and is commonly seen in IV drug abusers and those who had blood transfusions infected with the virus.
    - The disease is usually insidious in its presentation, and the severity is variable.

- As many as 50% of these patients may develop chronic disease, which may eventually lead to cirrhosis.
- The diagnosis is made by serologic means, and pegylated α-interferon and ribavirin have been used for treatment.

- *Hepatitis D:*

  - Also known as delta agent, it may coexist with hepatitis B.
  - It is usually associated with a more severe case of hepatitis B and cases of chronic hepatitis B in which there is reactivation of the virus.

- *Hepatitis E:*

  - The transmission is similar to the hepatitis A virus.
  - It is associated with a high fatality in pregnant women.

Pulmonary Tuberculosis

- Pulmonary TB refers to the clinical syndrome associated with infection of the respiratory system caused by *Mycobacterium tuberculosis*.
- M. tuberculosis is spread through the air from one person to another when bacteria are aerosolized from a person with pulmonary TB.
- Risk factors include:

    o HIV infection, substance abuse, DM, silicosis, cancer of the head or neck, leukemia or Hodgkin lymphoma, severe kidney disease, low body weight, certain treatments (e.g., corticosteroids), and recent immigration from a country with high rates of TB.

- Clinical features:

    o Most common symptom of pulmonary TB is productive cough for > 2 weeks.
    o May also have other respiratory symptoms (dyspnea, chest pain, hemoptysis) and/or constitutional symptoms (loss of appetite, weight loss, fever, night sweats, malaise).

- Diagnosis:

    o Suspect pulmonary TB in patients with suggestive symptoms of TB.
    o The classic chest radiography findings are cavitary upper lobe infiltrates, though infiltrates may appear anywhere in the lungs.
    o The presence of acid-fast bacilli (AFB) on a sputum sample smear usually indicates TB.

       ▪ Sputum samples should be at least 3, preferably in the early morning.

- o Additional findings that support the diagnosis if TB include a positive tuberculin skin test or interferon-gamma release assay (these tests do not distinguish latent from the active disease).
- o Rapid nucleic acid amplification testing with an Xpert Mycobacterium tuberculosis/rifampin (MTB/RIF) automated molecular test may be used to make a diagnosis or rule out a need for hospital airborne isolation in patients with suspected pulmonary TB.

- Management:

    - o Place hospitalized patients with suspected TB or who have an AFB smear-positive sputum airborne infection in isolation with appropriate infection control measures for providers and visitors.
    - o The recommended empiric treatment for pulmonary TB is a 2-month initial phase followed by a 4-month continuation phase.
    - o The 2-month initial phase consists of:

        - Isoniazid (PO, IV, or IM 5 mg/kg/day (maximum 300 mg/day, 10 mg/kg/day in children).
        - Rifampin (PO or IV 10 mg/kg/day (maximum 600 mg/day, 15 mg/kg/day in children).
        - Pyrazinamide (PO 25 mg/kg/day (maximum 2 g/day, 15-30 mg/kg/day in children).
        - Ethambutol (PO 15 mg/kg/day (maximum 1.6 g/day, 20 mg/kg/day in children).

    - o The 4-month continuation phase consists of:

        - Isoniazid.
        - Rifampin.

    - o Supplement the isoniazid treatment with pyridoxine (vitamin B6) 25 mg/day in patients with nutritional deficiency, diabetes, HIV infection, renal failure, or alcoholism, in pregnant and breastfeeding women, and in children to prevent adverse events.

- Repeat sputum cultures after the completion of the initial phase of the treatment.
- If cavities are present on an initial chest radiograph and if a culture of a specimen obtained at 2 months remains positive, extend the continuation phase to 7 months (9 months total).

Influenza

- Influenza infection is seasonal in temperate countries, with peaks during the winter months, but it has sustained activity throughout the year in tropical climates.
- Influenza is a single-stranded RNA virus, and member of the Orthomyxoviridae family.
- Infection can be caused by 1 of 3 types, subtypes A, B, and C:

  o Influenza A and B are the dominant circulating viruses.
  o Influenza A can be further classified based on 2 surface proteins: hemagglutinin (H) and neuraminidase (N).
  o Influenza C is believed to cause mild infection but does not contribute to seasonal epidemics.

- Transmission occurs via respiratory droplets and fomites. The incubation period is 1-4 days.
- Risk factors for complicated or severe disease course include:

  o Advanced age $\geq$ 65 years old or young age < 5 years.
  o Pregnancy.
  o Chronic conditions, including:

    - Pulmonary disease such as asthma or COPD.
    - DM.
    - Chronic cardiovascular, hepatic, renal, or hematologic disease.
    - Immunocompromise, including transplantation or immune suppressive drug regimens.
    - Morbid obesity.

- Clinical features include:

    o High fever, chills, myalgias and malaise, particularly in the winter months.

- Clinical diagnosis based on symptoms alone without lab testing can be made when influenza prevalence is high.
- Perform lab testing when result will change management of patients or contacts.

    o Multiple testing methods are available including rapid antigen detection tests (RADTS), reverse transcriptase-polymerase chain reaction (RT-PCR), and viral culture.

        - RADTS are fast and easy to perform, although negative result does not exclude influenza.
        - RT-PCR associated with high sensitivity compared to other tests, and can be used to verify negative rapid tests.

- Management:

    o Supportive care is the mainstay of treatment for most patients.
    o For high-risk patients or any patient with a severe clinical presentation, start neuraminidase inhibitors as soon as possible. Regimens include:

        - Oseltamivir 75 mg orally twice daily for 5 days.
        - Zanamivir 10 mg (2 inhalations) twice daily for 5 days.
        - Peramivir 600 mg IV single dose.

    o Oseltamivir and Zanamivir are approved for prophylaxis.
    o For antiviral agents to be effective, they must be initiated within 48 hours of the inset of influenza symptoms.
    o Antiviral agents reduce the duration of fever and illness by 1 day and also reduce the severity of some symptoms.

- Prevention:

    o Annual immunization is recommended for all individuals 6 months or older without contraindications.

- Major complications include primary influenza pneumonia and secondary bacterial pneumonia.

Dengue Fever

- Dengue is an acute febrile illness due to dengue virus (an arbovirus, member of the Flaviviridae, genus Flavivirus) infection and transmitted by Aedes mosquitoes bite.
- Classifications based on virulence of dengue genotypes:

  o DENV-1 and DENV-4 appear to be associated milder disease.
  o DENV-2 and DENV-3 appear to be associated with severe disease.

- Infection may be asymptomatic or present as a mild, self-limited febrile illness in most patients.
- A minority of patients may progress to severe disease, which may be characterized by as:

  o Plasma leakage, potentially progressive to shock.
  o Hemorrhage.
  o Severe organ impairment.
  o Dengue shock syndrome.

- Symptoms that are warning signs for developing severe dengue include:

  o Abdominal pain.
  o Persistent vomiting.
  o Mucosal bleeding (e.g. epistaxis).
  o Hepatomegaly.
  o Fluid accumulation in physical examination.
  o Lethargy or restlessness.

- Clinical Features:

- Fever (typically 4 to 10 days after exposure).
- Nausea/vomiting.
- Rash (typically begins as generalized or flushing erythema, later followed by maculopapular or morbilliform eruption.
- Aches and pains.

- Evaluation:

  - Common laboratory findings include leukopenia, thrombocytopenia, and elevated hematocrit.
  - Laboratory confirmation can be made using:

    - Viral cell culture.
    - Nucleic acid amplification tests (NAATs).
    - Serology.
    - Dengue antigen testing.

- The tourniquet test is part of WHO case definition and may aid in early diagnosis:

  - The test is performed by inflating the blood pressure cuff on the upper arm to a pressure midway between systolic and diastolic pressures and keeping that pressure in steady for 5 minutes.
  - The test is considered positive if > 20 petechiae are present per 2.5 cm^2 patch of skin on the forearm.

- Management:

  - Supportive care is the mainstay of treatment and is focused on:

    - Oral or IV fluid resuscitation, depending on severity of illness.
    - RBC transfusion if hemorrhagic complications.
    - Acetaminophen as pain reliever (avoid aspirin or other NSAIDs because of the risk of bleeding).

- Hospitalize patients with probable dengue with warning signs, patients with comorbidities, patients with severe disease, and patients unable to stay hydrated with oral intake.

Tetanus

- Tetanus is a vaccine-preventable, neurologic illness mediated by toxins produced by the soil-dwelling, anaerobic bacterium, Clostridium *tetani*.
- The illness typically manifests as one of 4 clinical syndromes:

  o Generalized tetanus, the most common form, is characterized by diffuse muscle spasms and rigidity.
  o Localized tetanus is characterized by pain and muscle spasms limited to the site of bacterial inoculation.
  o Cephalic tetanus is rare and typically manifests with cranial nerve palsies, resembling Bell palsy, or trigeminal neuritis.
  o Neonatal tetanus refers to generalized tetanus occurring in neonates born to mother who lack immunity.

- The source of illness is typically due to the contamination of a wound with C. *tetani* or inoculation of the organism into tissue, such as with penetrating trauma, IV drug use, or with unhygienic delivery conditions.
- Symptoms generally arise about 8 days after exposure, but the incubation period ranges from 3 to 21 days.
- Consider the diagnosis of tetanus in patients with no or unknown history of tetanus toxoid vaccination.
- Clinically compatible signs or symptoms such as:

  o Trismus (lockjaw).
  o Risus sardonicus (a characteristic facial expression arising from spasm of the facial muscle).
  o Generalized muscle spasm and rigidity.

- Characteristic facial expression with:

  o Raised eyebrows.

- o Tight closure of eyelids.
- o Wrinkling of forehead.
- o Extension of corners of mouth laterally.

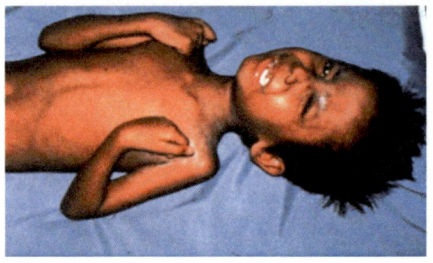

- The diagnosis is usually based on clinical findings and the exclusion of other disorders resembling tetanus such as drug-induced dystonias, trismus due to oral infections, hypocalcemia tetany, and strychnine poisoning.
- Management:

  - o Aggressive supportive care with admission to an intensive care unit may be needed for close monitoring and airway management.
  - o For those with wounds, provide appropriate wound care or debridement of any necrotic tissue, which may help reduce the bacterial and toxin burden at the inoculation site.
  - o Consider the use of antibiotics:

    - Metronidazole 500 mg IV or orally every 6 hours for 5-10 days in adults.

  - o To neutralize circulating tetanus toxin, consider antitetanus immunoglobulin, given as a single 500 unit intramuscular dose of human tetanus immune globulin (TIG) for adult patients.
  - o For the control of muscle spasms consider the use of a benzodiazepine, such as diazepam, midazolam, or lorazepam. Phenobarbital may be used when benzodiazepine not available.
  - o Magnesium sulfate, given as a continuous infusion, may also help reduce both muscle spasms and autonomic dysfunction. Other options include Labetalol, morphine, or clonidine.

- Prevention:

- Vaccinate all children without contraindications aged > 6 weeks and other persons with no or an incomplete vaccination history.
- Standard recommendation is a 5-dose immunization series beginning at age 3 months using (DTaP) vaccine.
- Provide a booster dose every 10 years.

Pertussis

- Pertussis, also known as Whooping cough, is a respiratory illness caused by *Bordetella pertussis*.
- Lack of immunity is a major risk factor for acquisition with populations most affected, including:

    o Infants < 6 months old, who are at risk for complications and severe disease.
    o Unvaccinated children.

- Illness occurs in 3 stages:

    o Catarrhal phase (1st phase, lasts 1-2 weeks):

        ▪ Non-specific prodromal symptoms (e.g. coryza, rhinorrhea, mild cough, fever).

    o Paroxysmal phase (2nd phase, lasts 4-6 weeks in children, up to 2-3 months in adults):

        ▪ Cough becomes spasmodic.
        ▪ Inspiration may produce characteristic "whoop", it's more common in children because of smaller tracheal diameter.

    o Convalescent phase (3rd phase, lasts 1-2 weeks):

        ▪ Associated with gradual decrease in cough frequency and severity.

- Evaluation:

- Patient may complain of:
    - Prolonged cough > 2 weeks, Paroxysms of coughing, Inspiratory "whoop".
    - Post-tussive vomiting.

- Diagnosis is confirmed with positive culture of B. pertussis, or positive PCR on nasopharyngeal sample (swab or aspirate).
- Management:
    - Macrolides are first line therapy. Azithromycin is commonly used and dosed as follows:
        - For infants < 6 months old, 10 mg/kg/day for 5 days.
        - For children > 6 months old, 10 mg/kg/day (maximum 500 mg) on day 1, then 5 mg/kg/day (maximum 250 mg) on days 2-5.
        - For adults, 500 mg on day 1, then 250 mg/day on days 2-5.
    - Clarithromycin or erythromycin can be used as alternatives for patients aged > 1 month.

- Hospitalization may be required especially in infants < 6 months old, for respiratory complications, leukocytosis with associated cardiopulmonary compromise, and feeding difficulties.
- Infection control measures include:
    - Use same antibiotics and dosing for treatment and post-exposure prophylaxis.
    - School or work exclusion for 5 days after the start of antibiotics.

Brucellosis

- Brucellosis (also called undulant fever, Malta fever) is caused by one of several species of the *Brucella* genus, most often *Brucella melitensis*.
- Risk factors include:

  o Persons with occupational exposure to animals are at increased risk, dairy industry workers, farmers, veterinarians, and microbiology laboratory personnel.

- Causes:

  o Ingestion of contaminated food is the most common source of transmission, particularly unpasteurized dairy products such as camel's milk and soft cheeses.
  o Consumption of undercooked meat products.

- Illness may be acute or insidious with symptoms typically arising 2-4 weeks after infection.
- Clinical features include:

  o A non-specific febrile illness is the most common manifestation, chills, malaise, headache, weight loss, lymphadenopathy, and hepatosplenomegaly.
  o Osteoarticular disease, such as arthritis, spondylitis, or osteomyelitis, is the most common site-specific.

- Diagnosis:

- A definitive diagnosis is made by a culture of blood, bone marrow, or other involved site.
- Serology may be useful when the organism can't be cultured or a culture is not available.

- **Management:**

  - Antibiotic therapy should be initiated in all cases, even in those spontaneously improving.
  - Tetracyclines, such as doxycycline, are the backbone of therapy.
  - Due to high rates of relapse, Tetracyclines are given in combination with a second active agent, such as an aminoglycoside.
    - Doxycycline plus rifampicin is an option.
  - Uncomplicated brucellosis (without focal infection) is typically treated for 6 weeks.
  - Management of complicated cases will vary based on the site of involvement, but antibiotic therapy may be needed for 8 weeks or longer.
  - Without treatment, acute infection may progress to chronic illness persisting for years.
  - With treatment, relapse occurs in 4-24% and varies with the treatment regimen used.

Malaria

- Malaria is a systemic infection of erythrocytes by plasmodia protozoa (*Plasmodium falciparum* is most commonly), transmitted to humans through bites of infected mosquitoes.
- Uncomplicated malaria (caused by *P. falciparum, P. vivax, P. ovale, P. malaria*).
- Severe malaria (usually caused by *P. falciparum*).
- Clinical features include:

    o Fever, vomiting, headaches, chills, muscle aches, anorexia.
    o Dark or red urine due to the presence of hemoglobin and myoglobin.
    o Look for a traveler recently returning from an endemic area.

- Diagnosis:

    o In low-risk settings, suspect malaria if both:

        - Possibility of exposure to malaria
        - History of fever in previous 3 days with no features of other severe disease.

    o In high-risk settings, suspect malaria if either:

        - History of fever in previous 24 hours.
        - Anemia (pallor of palms appears to be most reliable sign in young children).

    o Prompt parasitologic diagnosis for confirmation recommended in all patients suspected of malaria before starting treatment (if possible), using either microscopy or rapid diagnostic tests (RDT):

- Identifiable parasites on light microscopy of thick and thin blood smears.
- RDT of *Plasmodium* antigen.

- Management:

  o Treatment of uncomplicated P. falciparum malaria:

  - Artemisinin-based combination therapy (ACT) is effective. Choice of ACT based on level of resistance in region. ACT should include at least 3 days of treatment with an Artemisinin derivative.
  - ACTs should be used in preference to sulfadoxine-pyrimethamine (SP) plus amodiaquine (AQ) for treatment of uncomplicated P. falciparum malaria.
  - <u>Specific regimen include</u>: (Artemether + Lumefantrine), (Artesunate + Amodiaquine), (Artesunate + Mefloquine).

  o Dihydroartemisinin plus Piperaquine (DHA + PPQ) is an option for 1st-line treatment of uncomplicated P. falciparum malaria worldwide.

  o Second-line antimalarial treatments include:

  - Artesunate plus tetracycline, doxycycline, or clindamycin for 7 days.
  - Quinine plus tetracycline, doxycycline, or clindamycin for 7 days.

  o Recommendations for pregnant women in 1st TRIMESTER:

  - Quinine + clindamycin for 7 days.
  - Artesunate + clindamycin for 7 days (INDICATED IF ABOVE REGIMEN FAILED).
  - ACTs indicated only if ACT is the only treatment immediately available, if quinine + clindamycin fails, or compliance with 7-day treatment uncertain.

- Recommendations for pregnant women in 2nd or 3rd TRIMESTER:

    - ACTs known to be effective.
    - Artesunate + clindamycin for 7 days.

- For lactating women:

    - Use standard antimalarial treatment (including ACTs) except for Dapsone, Primaquine, and Tetracycline.

- For infants and young children, use ACT as 1st-line treatment.
- For travelers returning to non-endemic countries, prophylaxis options include:

    - Atovaquone-Proguanil.
    - Artemether-Lumefantrine.
    - Quinine plus doxycycline or clindamycin.

- Therapeutic dose ranges:

    - Artesunate 2-10 mg/kg/day
    - Lumefantrine 10-16 mg/kg/day
    - Amodiaquine 7.5-15 mg/kg/day
    - Mefloquine 7-11 mg/kg/day

Chickenpox

- Chickenpox is a highly contagious illness caused by primary infection with the varicella zoster virus, characterized by vesicular rash and fever.
- Incubation period typically 14-16 days (range from 10 to 21 days).
- Chickenpox typically presents in children.
- In infants, adults, and immunocompromised patients, symptoms may be more severe.
- Clinical features include:

    o Vesicular pruritic rash, which usually begins on the head and trunk with subsequent lesions on extremities.
    o Crops of lesions at various stages may be present together.
    o New lesion form for up to 1 week, with the total number of vesicles usually 250-500.
    o Lesions develop crust with hypopigmentation in final stages.
    o In adults and immunocompromised (prolonged fever, more lesions, and pneumonia).

- Differential diagnosis includes: (scabies, erythema multiforme, contact dermatitis).
- Management:

    o In otherwise healthy children < 12 years old, treatment is symptom-directed and antiviral medication is usually not needed.
    o Give Acyclovir (or other antiviral drug) for immunocompromised patients, patients with chronic skin or lung disease, severe cases of varicella, neonatal varicella, adults, and pregnant women.
    o Use varicella zoster immune globulin (VariZIG) as post-exposure prophylaxis in immunocompromised patients, pregnant women, premature infants, and neonates born to mothers with evidence of

infection if able to give within 96 hours of exposure to varicella (preferably within 48 hours).

- Prevention:

    o Varicella virus vaccine is recommended to prevent chickenpox in adults and children > 12 months old, unless immunocompromised.

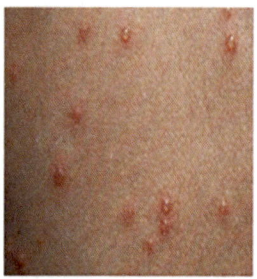 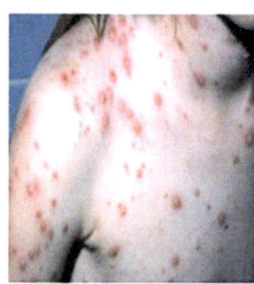 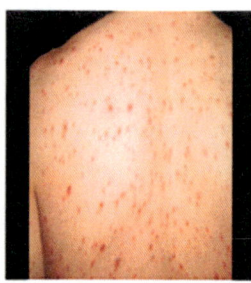

Infectious Mononucleosis

- Infectious mononucleosis, also known as kissing disease, or glandular fever, is an infection usually caused by the Epstein-Barr virus.
- The virus spreads through saliva, which is why it's sometimes called kissing disease.
- Risk factors include:

  o Day care centers, residence in developing nations, poor sanitary conditions, kissing, other settings in which exchange of saliva or oropharyngeal secretions may be likely.

- Clinical features include:

  o Over 80% of patients present with the classic triad of:

    - Fever.
    - Pharyngitis.
    - Lymphadenopathy, most often posterior cervical.

  o Additional common symptoms include fatigue, malaise, headache, abdominal pain, nausea, vomiting, or rash.
  o Heaviness or fullness in left upper quadrant may suggest splenic enlargement.
  o Significant left upper quadrant abdominal pain or severe left shoulder tip pain (Kehr sign) may indicate splenic rupture.

- Diagnosis:
  o Consider heterophile antibody testing (such as Monospot) within the first several weeks of illness to confirm the diagnosis.

- This test is highly specific in patients with clinically compatible syndromes, but the sensitivity varies with the patient age, test used, and time since the illness onset.

    o When heterophile antibody testing is negative, consider EBV-specific serologies for a definitive diagnosis.

- Management:

    o Supportive care is the mainstay of treatment.

        - Acetaminophen or NSAIDs for fever and sore throat. Adequate fluid intake to avoid dehydration.

    o Antiviral therapy is NOT recommended for routine use.
    o Corticosteroids are NOT recommended for routine use, but may be used when there is concern for complications such as airway obstruction.
    o Consider activity restriction for a minimum of 3 weeks to avoid splenic rupture

Oral Candidiasis

- Oral candidiasis, also called thrush, is the most common fungal infection in humans.
- Candida *albicans* is the most common cause.
- Risk factors include:

    o Immunocompromised, particularly HIV infection, corticosteroid use, antibiotic use, nutritional deficiencies, denture use, and extremes of age.

- Signs and symptoms associated with thrush include oral discomfort and the development of whitish plaques on the tongue or oral mucosa.

    o Lesions that easily bleed and can be scraped away with a tongue depressor.

- Diagnosis is typically made based on compatible clinical features.
- Differential diagnosis:

    o Lichen planus, Psoriasis, Erythema multiforme, Oral hairy leukoplakia.
    o Group A streptococcus infection resulting in scarlet fever.
    o Nutritional deficiencies such as Vitamin B3 and B 12 deficiency.
    o Herpes simplex esophagitis.

- When needed, clinical diagnosis can be confirmed by:

    o Potassium chloride (KOH) or Calcofluor stain of swab or scraping from affected area.
    o Fungal culture of swab, scraping, or oral rinse.

- Management:

    o Encourage good oral hygiene such as tooth-brushing, routine dentistry, and denture care.
    o First-line regimens for mild disease include topical agents such as:

        - Clotrimazole troches 10 mg orally 5 times daily for 7-14 days.

    o Systemic therapy is recommended for all moderate and severe cases.

        - Fluconazole 100-200 mg orally once daily is the 1st line therapy.
        - The recommended duration of therapy is 7-14 days.

- For fluconazole-refractory disease, consider:

    o Itraconazole 200 mg orally once daily for up to 28 days.
    o Posaconazole initially 400 mg orally twice daily for 3 days, then 400 mg daily for up to 28 days.

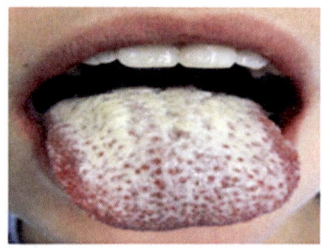 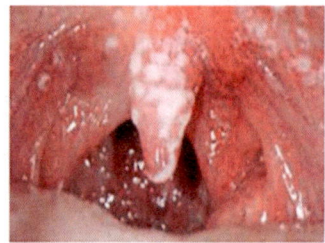

Fever of Unknown Origin

- Key features of fever of unknown origin (FUO), also known as pyrexia of unknown origin (PUO):

  o Temperature greater than 38.3°C on several occasions.
  o More than 3 weeks' duration of illness.
  o Failure to reach a diagnosis despite one week of inpatient investigation.

- FUO is classified into 4 categories:

  o Classic FUO.
  o Hospital-acquired FUO.
  o Immunocompromised or neutropenic FUO.
  o HIV-related FUO.

- Etiology includes:

  o Infectious causes of FUO:

    - *Most common*: Tuberculosis, Q fever, Brucellosis.
    - *Less common*: HIV infection, abdominopelvic abscesses, Cat scratch disease, EBV infection, CMV infection, Enteric fever, Toxoplasmosis.
    - *Least common*: Subacute bacterial endocarditis (SBE), Tooth abscess, Sinusitis.

  o Non-infectious inflammatory causes of FUO (Connective tissue diseases, Vasculitides, and Granulomatous disorders):
    - Most common: Giant cell (temporal) arteritis, Adult Still disease (juvenile RA).

- Less common: SLE, Periarteritis nodosa/microscopic polyangiitis (PAN/MPA), RA.
- Least common: Antiphospholipid syndrome (APS), Gout, Bechet disease, Sarcoidosis, Felty syndrome, Takayasu arteritis, Kikuchi disease.

o Malignant and neoplastic causes of FUO:

- *Most common*: Lymphoma, renal cell carcinoma.
- *Less common*: Myeloproliferative disorder, acute myelogenous leukemia.
- *Least common*: Multiple myeloma, beast/liver/pancreatic/colon cancer, atrial myxoma, metastases to brain/liver/ malignant histiocytosis.

o Miscellaneous causes of FUO:

- *Most common*: Cirrhosis (due to portal endotoxins), Drug fever.
- *Less common*: Thyroiditis, Crohn disease (regional enteritis).
- *Least common*: PE, hypothalamic syndrome, and familial periodic syndromes.

- Clinical features include:

o The history can provide important clues to FUO.
o In general, specific fever patterns do not correlate strongly with specific diseases.
o Definitive documentation of fever and exclusion of factitious fever are essential early steps in the physical examination.
o Tenderness to percussion over a vertebra (vertebral osteomyelitis, TB, typhoid, brucellosis).
o Splenomegaly without hepatomegaly (bacterial endocarditis, EBV/CMV infection, TB, histoplasmosis, brucellosis, malaria, cirrhosis).

- Diagnosis:

    o CBC, peripheral blood smear, chemistry, blood cultures, HIV serology, TB screening tests, ESR.
    o Imaging should be directed by historical, physical, and basic laboratory clues.
    o Some procedures such as endoscopy and biopsies may be needed.

- Management:

    o In general, empiric therapy has little or no role in cases of classic FUO.
    o Treatment should be directed toward the underlying cause, as needed, once a diagnosis is made.
    o No evidence supports prolonged hospitalization of patients who are clinically stable and whose workup findings are unrevealing.
    o Conduct close follow-up procedures and systematic reevaluation studies to prevent clinical worsening.
    o The choice of medications administered to patients depends on the etiology of the FUO.

Section 9: Musculoskeletal

Acute Low Back Pain

- Nonspecific acute low back pain is a diagnosis of exclusion.
- Acute low back pain (LBP) is nonspecific pain lasting < 6 weeks. Subacute back pain lasts 6 weeks to 3 months. Back pain lasting > 3 months is considered chronic low back pain.
- Causes:

  o Most cases are idiopathic, often presumed to be nonspecific lumbar strain.
  o Specific mechanical causes of low back pain include (herniated disk, degenerative joint disease of the low back, vertebral fracture, spinal stenosis, spondylolisthesis, kyphosis, scoliosis).
  o All nonmechanical causes (such as cancer, osteomyelitis, etc.) account for about 1% of cases.

- Evaluation:

  o Evaluate the patient's history and physical exam for signs or symptoms of radiculopathy, spinal stenosis, malignancy, infection, cauda equina syndrome, vertebral fracture, ankylosing spondylitis, severe or progressive motor neuron disease, and herniated disc.
  o Do not routinely obtain imaging studies or other diagnostic tests in patients with nonspecific low back pain.
  o Perform diagnostic imaging and testing only for patients with severe or progressive neurologic deficits or suspected of having serious underlying conditions. "Red flag" findings that are indications for imaging include:

- Onset at age < 20 years or > 55 years.
- Pain that is unrelenting at night, unrelated to time or activity (nonmechanical), or thoracic.
- Neurologic exam findings of nerve root compression.

  o Use MRI or CT if vertebral infection or cauda equina syndrome are suspected, if severe or progressive neurologic deficits are present, or if symptoms are suggestive of radiculopathy (from either spinal stenosis or herniated disc) despite adequate period of conservative therapy.

- Management:

  o Advice patients with nonspecific LBP to remain active and to return to normal activities as soon as symptoms allow.
  o Consider heat therapy for short-term pain reduction.
  o Provide patient education on LBP including expected course and advice to remain active.
  o If using medications for LBP:

    - Acetaminophen, NSAIDs, Muscle relaxants, Opioid analgesia are the preferred options.

Osteoarthritis

- It is a common degenerative disorder of the articular cartilage associated with hypertrophic changes.
- The joints most commonly affected are knees, hands, hips, and spine.
- It is classified based on joint distribution into:

    - *Localized OA:* when there is single joint is affected; it could be unilateral or bilateral.
    - *Generalized OA:* when there is OA at the spinal or hand joints, and at least two other joint regions.

- Risk factors include: Age, Obesity, Female gender, Occupation, Sports activities, Previous injury, Muscle weakness, and Proprioceptive deficits.
- Etiology of OA is either:

    - *Primary OA:* idiopathic, no preceding injury to the joint. It affects about 90% of patient with OA.
    - *Secondary OA:* when there is an antecedent insult to the joint such as congenital abnormality, trauma, infection (e.g. septic arthritis), and inflammatory arthropathies (e.g. Rheumatoid arthritis).

- Pathophysiology of OA include wearing away the articular cartilage by the risk factors, the exposed bony surfaces rubbed together, this, along with the grow of bony projections called bone spurs, cause swelling, pain and limited movements of the joints.
- Clinical manifestations of OA include:

    - Pain with joint use and relieved by rest.

- Pain in the knee OA may be anteromedial or more generalized on the medial side.

  - Morning stiffness for < 30 minutes.
  - Reduced range of motion.
  - Crepitation.
  - Bony deformity.

- Lab tests such as Rheumatoid factor, ESR, and CRP are normal.
- Synovial fluid analysis usually non-inflammatory or mildly inflammatory with less than 2000 WBCs/mm3, predominantly mononuclear cells.
- Findings on OA x-ray include:

  - Joint space narrowing.
  - Osteophytes.
  - Subchondral sclerosis.
  - Subchondral cysts.

- Non-pharmacological treatment include weight loss, exercise and physical therapy, rest for a short period 12-24 hours (avoid complete rest because it may lead to a loss of muscle and joint stiffness), orthoses, braces, or assistive devices may be used, oral glucosamine and chondroitin are not recommended.
- Pharmacological treatment include:

  - The *first line therapy* is local analgesia such as topical NSAIDs (Diclofenac Sodium), Methylsalicylate Cream or Capsaicin. Side effects include mild skin rash (NSAIDs) and burning sensation (Capsaicin).
  - *Second line therapy* that relieves the pain (mild to moderate) but don't have effect in inflammation is Acetaminophen, 500-1000 mg PRN Q6hrs (maximum 4000 mg/day).
  - *Third line therapy* that reduces inflammation and relives the pain (moderate to severe) is NSAIDs, Ibuprofen 400-800 mg Q8hrs, or

Meloxicam 7.5-15 mg OD. Avoid NSAIDs in patients with renal insufficiency.
- *Fourth line therapy* is opioids, can relieve severe pain but don't have effect on inflammation, Codeine 15-60 mg Q6hrs (maximum 360 mg / day).
- *Injectable therapy* which suppress inflammation and can relieve severe symptoms are:

    - *Glucocorticoid injections:* recommended no more than 3 to 4 injections per year, the effect often lasted up to 8 weeks. For small joints 10 mg (e.g. MTP), 20 mg for medium-sized joints (e.g. wrists, elbow), and 40 mg for larger joints (e.g. knee, hip).
    - *Hyaluronate injections:* the treatment effect of hyaluronic acid often lasted for up to 4 months, the biggest drawback of hyaluronic acid injections is the cost.

- Surgery is recommended before arthritis cause complications such as muscle loss and joint deformities.

    - Options of surgery include joint replacement and osteotomy.

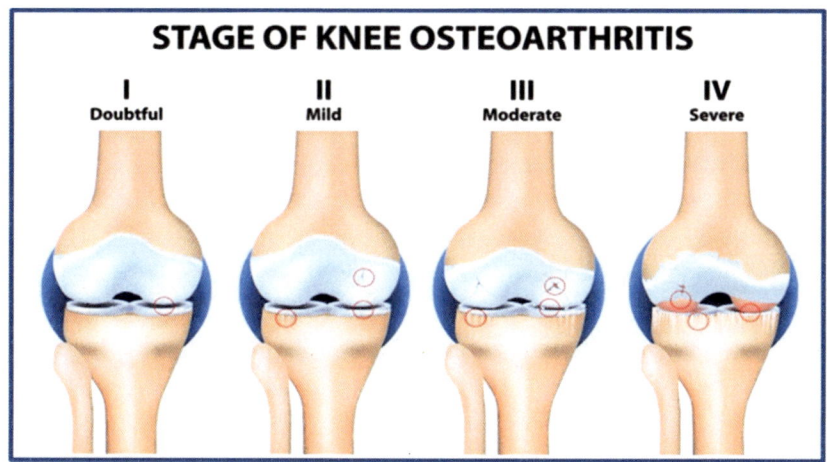

Osteoporosis

- It is a generalized skeletal disorder characterized by compromised bone strength and deterioration of bone quality, often leading to fragility fracture.
- Osteomalacia: is a softening of bones, usually due to severe lack of vitamin D.
- Risk factors:

  o Lifestyle factors (i.e. low calcium intake, vitamin D deficiency, inadequate physical activity, smoking, and alcohol abuse).
  o Certain endocrine (e.g. DM, hyperparathyroidism, Cushing syndrome), GI (e.g. Celiac disease, gastric bypass, malabsorption), hematologic (multiple myeloma, thalassemia, mastocytosis), autoimmune, and CNS disorders increases the risk.
  o Medications such as: long-term anticoagulation, hormonal therapies, glucocorticosteriods, some immunosuppressants, lithium, thiazolidinediones (glitazone), and long-term PPI use may also cause osteoporosis.
  o Postmenopausal women.
  o Persons > 65 years old.
  o Persons with small body frame.

- Classifications:

  o Primary osteoporosis:

    - Deterioration of bone mass unassociated with other chronic illness, related to aging and decreased gonadal function (bone loss accelerated during sixth decade of life or perimenopausal period in women).

- - Secondary osteoporosis:
    - Deterioration of bone mass associated with chronic conditions that contribute significantly to accelerated bone loss.

- Pathophysiology:
  - In healthy bone, bone resorption (osteoclast cells) is balanced by bone formation (osteoblast cells).
  - Bone loss occurs when bone resorption outpaces bone formation, resulting in decreased bone mass and increased risk of fracture.
  - Fracture results from overloading of weakened bones.

- Clinical features:
  - Patients usually asymptomatic until fracture.
  - Fractures most likely to be due to osteoporosis include:
    - Femoral neck fractures, Pathologic fractures of vertebra, Lumbar and thoracic vertebral fractures, distal radius fractures.
  - Back pain and postural change may occur with vertebral fractures.

- Diagnosis:
  - The diagnosis is made in adults with fragility fracture, regardless of any test results.
  - If no fragility fracture, consider screening for osteoporosis with bone mineral density testing (usually Dual-Energy X-Ray Absorptiometry measurement DEXA at posterior-anterior spine and hip).
  - Osteoporosis is defined as a fragility fracture or T-score < 2.5 when determined by lowest calculation from lumbar spine (at least 2 evaluable vertebra), femoral neck, or total femur T-score.

- Osteopenia is low normal bone density that is not low enough to be osteoporosis, as defined by T-score between -1 and -2.5 when determined by lowest calculation from lumbar spine, femoral neck, or total femur.

CLASSIFICATION OF T-SCORE BASED ON WHO INTERNATIONAL CLASSIFICATION:

T-Score	Interpretation
> -1	Normal
-1 to -2.5	Low bone mass (Osteopenia)
< -2.5	Osteoporosis
T-score < -2.5 and > 1 fractures	Severe or established osteoporosis

- Management:
  - Encourage all patients with osteoporosis or increased risk of osteoporosis to initiate lifestyle changes including (balanced diet with adequate calcium and vitamin D intake, regular weight-bearing and muscle-strengthening exercise, and smoking cessation).
  - Select Bisphosphonate as 1st-line therapy for most patients.
    - Such as Alendronate 10 mg or Risedronate 5 mg orally once daily.
  - Parathyroid hormone 1-34 (teriparatide) 20 mcg subcutaneously once daily can be 1st-line choice for patients at highest risk for fractures.

Scaphoid Fracture

- Fracture of the scaphoid, the carpal bone articulating with distal radius, trapezium, and capitate.
- It is most common in young males age 15-30 years.
- Scaphoid fracture results from fall on outstretched hand (FOOSH) or forced wrist extension.
- The pathogenesis includes falling on extended, radially deviated wrist cause extreme dorsiflexion and compression to radial side of hand.
- The presenting complaint is usually deep dull pain in wrist worsened by gripping or squeezing.
- High clinical suspicion of occult scaphoid fracture if all of following 3 criteria seen:

    o Tenderness on palpation of anatomic snuff box.
    o Tenderness on axial loading for first ray.
    o Swelling at anatomic snuff box.

- Moderate clinical suspicion if 2 criteria, low clinical suspicion if 1 criterion.
- Clinical exam not accurate for detecting occult scaphoid fracture.
- Special tests include:

    o *Watson's test (i.e., Scaphoid shift test):*

        ▪ Tenderness and popping of scaphoid bone felt over volar wrist during radial and ulnar deviation or wrist.

    o *Scaphoid compression test:*

- ■ Compress patient's thumb axially/longitudinally along first metacarpal, found to be able to identify source of scaphoid fracture even when a cast is in place.

- Differential diagnosis include:

    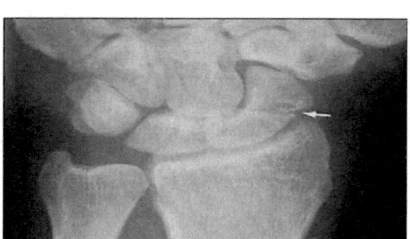

    o Fracture of other metacarpal bones or distal radius.
    o Arthritis of carpometacarpal or radiocarpal joint.
    o De Quervain's Tenosynovitis.
    o Extensor carpi radialis strain.

- Imaging studies to confirm diagnosis include:

    o *X-Ray:* especially scaphoid view "oblique" (wrist is ulnar-deviated and extended while film is shot dorsal-volar view).
    o *MRI:* is considered when scaphoid fracture suspected and x-ray is negative.
    o Bone scintigraphy, Ultrasound, and CT.

- Management include:

    o *For suspected fracture with initial negative x-ray:* consider casting for 2 weeks and reevaluation.
    o *Non-displaced fracture:* cast immobilization is recommended.
    o *Displaced fracture:* splinting and referral to orthopedic, also for non-displaced proximal or medial fractures because of displacement risk.

- Complications include:

    o Delayed union.
    o Decreased grip strength.
    o Decreased range of motion.
    o Osteoarthritis.

Gout

- Gout and pseudogout are the 2 most common crystal-induced arthropathies.
- Gout is caused by monosodium urate monohydrate crystals.
- Pseudogout is caused by calcium pyrophosphate crystals and is more accurately termed calcium pyrophosphate disease.
- Risk factors include:

    o Obesity, HTN, high consumption of alcohol or high-purine foods, and several types of antihypertensive medications including diuretics, beta blockers.

- Clinical features include:

    o Typically, there are 4 stages of disease progression:

    - Asymptomatic, acute, intercritical, and chronic.

    o Episodes of acute gout are characterized by severe pain, erythema, warmth, and swelling of one or more joints, peaking within 24-48 hours and with spontaneous resolution within 3-14 days.
    o The 1st metatarsophalangeal joint is most commonly affected. Other frequently involved joints include the midfoot, ankles, and knees.
    o The disease may ultimately progress to chronic tophaceous gout with persistent arthritis, white-yellow intradermal deposits, and frequent recurrent acute attacks.

- Diagnosis:

- The gold standard for diagnosis is demonstration of urate crystals (needle shaped with strong negative birefringence) in synovial fluid or tophus by polarized light microscopy.
- Testing may include serum uric acid level (although it has limited usefulness during an acute attack), CBC, BUN, creatinine, and imaging such as X-ray, ultrasound, or CT.

- Differential diagnosis include:

  - Septic arthritis, bacterial cellulitis, rheumatoid arthritis, psoriatic arthritis, erosive OA.

- Management:

  - For acute attacks:

    - Usually self-limited with complete and spontaneous resolution in 3-13 days.
    - Non-pharmacological treatment includes rest, ice packs, and elevation of affected joints.
    - For attacks with mild-to-moderate pain affecting 1-2 joints, use monotherapy as:

      - Indomethacin (NSAIDs) 50 mg TID.
      - Naproxen 750 mg then 250 mg TID.
      - Low dose Colchicine 1.2 mg PO then 0.6 mg 1 hour later.
      - Prednisone 0.5 mg/kg once daily for 5-10 days.
      - Methylprednisolone 0.5-2 mg/kg IV or intramuscularly once.
      - Intra-articular corticosteroids injection has been reported to be effective.

  - For attacks with severe pain, especially if acute polyarticular involving multiple large joints:

- High dose Colchicine 1.2 mg PO followed by 0.6 mg hourly for 6 hours, plus NSAIDs.
- Systemic corticosteroid and high dose colchicine.
- Intra-articular corticosteroid with any other treatment.

o For prevention of recurrent attacks:

- Urate-lowering therapy is recommended for patients with gout and 2 or more attacks per year, tophi, a uric acid stone, or reduced kidney function.
- First line options include Xanthine oxidase inhibitors:

  ❖ Allopurinol 50-100 mg/day orally, titrated every few weeks until the target uric acid level is achieved, up to maximum 800-900 mg/day.
  ❖ Febuxostat 40-80 mg PO OD, although doses > 80 mg/day may increase risk of gout flare.

- Second line options in patients with normal renal function include agents such as:

  ❖ Probenecid, Sulfinpyrazone, or benzbromarone.

- For most patients, titrate urate-lowering therapy to a target serum uric acid level of < 6 mg/dL, although some patients may require a level of < 5 mg/dL to control symptoms.
- Continue urate-lowering therapy during an acute gout attack.
- If the patient is not currently receiving treatment, wait 1-2 weeks after inflammation has settled to start urate-lowering therapy.
- For patients on urate-lowering therapy, measure serum uric acid and creatinine levels every 3 months for the first year and then annually thereafte

Fibromyalgia

- Fibromyalgia is a chronic, non-inflammatory, diffuse pain disorder marked by widespread musculoskeletal pain.
- It is more common in women, especially middle age.
- The etiology is unknown.
- The disease course is generally chronic, although improvement in symptoms may occur in approximately 25% of even untreated patients over 2-3 years.
- Associated symptoms include:

    o Fatigue, sleep difficulty, cognitive dysfunction, and depressed mood or depressive episodes.

- Diagnosis:

    o Suspect fibromyalgia in patients with chronic diffuse pain that cannot be explained by other disorders.
    o Diagnose fibromyalgia in patient with diffuse symptoms not explained by other disorders for at least 3 months and have either:

    - Widespread pain index (WPI) $\geq$ 7 and symptom severity (SS) scale score $\geq$ 5 or WPI 3-6 and SS scale score $\geq$ 9
    - A history of pain on both sides of the body, above and below the waist and pain involving the neck, trunk, or low back, and pain on digital palpation of at least 11 tender points.

    o Lab test is not useful to make the diagnosis. Consider testing only to evaluate for other disorders.
- Management:

- Tailor treatment to the specific needs of each patient, which should include education, exercise activity and cognitive behavioral therapy.
- Consider pharmacologic management for specific symptoms. Combination therapy may be required. Options include:

  - Any antidepressant may be used to reduce pain, fatigue, and improve depressed mood in patients with fibromyalgia. Amitriptyline 25-50 mg at bedtime has the most evidence of efficacy.
  - Cyclobenzaprine 5-20 mg at bedtime may improve restorative sleep.
  - Pregabalin 150 mg/day to 450 mg/day in divided doses, or gabapentin 800-2400 mg/day in divided doses reduces pain and improves sleep.
  - Acetaminophen or NSAIDs to reduce pain, but prescribe at the lowest dose for the shortest time period due to possible serious adverse events.
  - Consider a low potency opioid such as tramadol only for patients with symptoms refractory to other treatments. Avoid high potency opioids.

Plantar Fasciitis

- It is a degenerative condition of the plantar fascia that results in heel pain with symptoms ranging from mild to severe.
- The exact cause is unknown but a common theory is repetitive micro-trauma from prolonged walking or running.
- The diagnosis should be made based on the clinical exam including the following history and PE:

    o Plantar medial heel pain (worse after a period of inactivity and with prolonged weight-bearing).
    o Heel pain following recent increase in weight-bearing activity.
    o Pain with palpation of proximal insertion of plantar fascia.
    o Positive windlass test.
    o Negative results on tests for tarsal tunnel syndrome.
    o Limited active and passive talocrural joint dorsiflexion range of motion.

- Initial management:

    o Use plantar-fascia-specific and gastrocnemius/soleus stretching for short term (1 week-4 months).
    o NSAIDs or acetaminophen to reduce pain.
    o Use anti-pronation taping (up to 3 weeks).
    o Use foot orthoses and heel pads/cups to support medial longitudinal arch and cushion heel.

Osteomyelitis

- Osteomyelitis is a bacterial or fungal infection of the bone.
- It may present as acute (evolving within days to 2 weeks) or chronic infection (presence of necrosis).
- *Staphylococcus aureus* is the most common pathogens.
- Risk factors include (open fracture, chronic soft tissue infection, use of IV drugs or catheter).
- Clinical features include:

    o Acute onset of fever with pain, erythema, and swelling at the affected site.
    o Chronic pain, persistent sinus tract or wound drainage, and soft tissue damage, particularly in patients with diabetes and peripheral vascular disease.

- Diagnosis:

    o Probe-to-bone test.
    o Blood test (may show leukocytosis, thrombocytosis, and elevated inflammatory markers).
    o X-ray (low sensitivity early in course), MRI, CT (useful for guiding a needle biopsy).
    o Definitive diagnosis of chronic osteomyelitis requires a bone biopsy for pathology and culture.

- Management:

- The duration of therapy is usually > 4-6 weeks. Broad-spectrum empiric antibiotics may be appropriate before receipt of culture (Vancomycin, Ceftriaxone, Cefazoline).
- A surgical approach may be required in patients with antibiotic failure, infected surgical hardware, or chronic osteomyelitis with necrotic bone and soft tissue.

Paronychia

- Paronychia is an inflammation of the tissue folds immediately surrounding a fingernail or toenail.
- Classifications:

  o Acute paronychia: is characterized by a duration of < 6 weeks and is most commonly caused by bacterial infection (*Staph. aureus*) following minor nail bed cuticle (proximal nail fold) trauma.

    - Nail biting or picking increase the risk of acute paronychia of the hands.
    - Ingrown toenails may increase the risk of acute paronychia of the feet.

  o Chronic paronychia: is characterized by a duration of > 6 weeks and is most commonly related to chronic exposure to environmental irritants or allergens.

    - Occupations associated with chronic paronychia include dishwashers, barbers, cooks, healthcare professionals, or other work requiring contact with moisture or irritants.
    - Cultures of chronic paronychia are frequently positive for Candida. Spp., but it is unclear if yeast is a causative agent or colonizer of underlying inflammation.

- Comorbidities such as diabetes or immunosuppression can increase the risk of paronychia.
- Certain medications are also associated paronychia as an adverse effect, including retinoids, and antiretroviral therapy with indinavir.

- Evaluation:

  - The diagnosis can be made based on clinical findings.
  - Physical exam shows swelling, erythema, and tenderness. Chronic paronychia may be associated with nail abnormalities, such as thickening, ridging, or discoloration.

- Differential diagnosis:

  - Herpetic whitlow, contact dermatitis, splinter or foreign body, psoriasis, as well as benign or malignant skin lesions.

- Testing is not usually needed to diagnose paronychia, but if the infection or abscess appears severe, consider obtaining a specimen of purulent material to rule out MRSA.

  - Consider X-ray of foreign body or trauma is suspected, or to screen for osteomyelitis.
  - Consider biopsy if any malignancy or systemic etiologies are suspected.

- Management:

  - For mild to moderate acute paronychia:

    - Warm soaks and topical antibiotics are usually sufficient to resolve the infection.
    - Consider topical steroids and NSAIDs to reduce pain and symptoms.
    - If the abscess is present, consider incision and drainage with a bacterial and viral culture of purulent material.

  - For more severe acute paronychia:

- Consider anti-staphylococcal oral antibiotics.
- If MRSA is prevalent in the area, consider Trimethoprim-Sulfamethoxazole.
- If the bacterial source is presumed to be oral flora, consider amoxicillin/clavulanate.

o For paronychia associated with ingrown toenails:

- Address the ingrown toenail of possible.

o For chronic paronychia:

- The mainstay of management is avoidance of moisture and irritants in an effort to reduce ongoing inflammation.
- Consider topical steroids, such as betamethasone.
- Consider a topical antifungal, such as ciclopirox, or ketoconazole.
- Consider surgical intervention for recalcitrant chronic paronychia that is unresponsive to the avoidance of irritants and topical or systemic medications.
- Surgical interventions aim to remove fibrotic tissue of the proximal nail fold to allow for improved blood flow and healing of chronic paronychia.

Section 10: Nephrology

Renal Stone

- Kidney stones (renal calculi) are crystalline mineral deposits that form in the kidney, and may occur in 1%-20% of people during their lifetime.
- Hypercalciuria is the most common underlying metabolic precipitant. Other causes include hyperoxaluria, hyperuricosuria, hypocitraturia, cystinuria, low urinary volume, UTI, and medications.
- Calcium (oxalate or phosphate) is the most common constituent of stones, with other common constituent being struvite (associated with infection) and uric acid.
- Estimated spontaneous passage rates are 68% for stones < 5 mm and 47% for stones 5-10 mm, but spontaneous passage may take more than 1 week.
- Evaluation:
    - Patients are often asymptomatic until a stone causes partial, intermittent, or complete obstruction, resulting in acute and debilitating renal colic.
    - Perform immediate imaging in patients in patients with fever or solitary kidney, or when the diagnosis of stones is in doubt.
        - For imaging of nephrolithiasis, noncontrast CT is a first-line imaging choice as it has the best sensitivity and specificity, but carries a significant radiation exposure.
        - US is an alternative first-line imaging test and is the best of choice in children, in pregnant women, and persons with a history of radio-opaque stones.
    - Obtain blood tests including serum creatinine, uric acid, and ionized calcium.
    - Obtain urinalysis and urine culture or microscopy to rule out infection. Consider obtaining two 24-hour urine collections as part

of a comprehensive metabolic evaluation for patients with or at risk for multiple stone episodes, including those with nephrocalcinosis.
- Obtain a stone composition analysis for the first stone that is able to be recovered.
- Conduct a full metabolic evaluation (informed by stone composition and including two 24-hour urine collections) in high-risk stone formers.
- Kidney-ureter-bladder (KUB) radiography can help to differentiate between radiolucent and radiopaque stones and be used for comparison during follow-up.

- Management:

  - Pain management:

    - Offer a NSAID (such as metamizol, diclofenac, indomethacin, or ibuprofen) as drug of first choice for initial pain control. Offer hydromorphone, pentazocine, or tramadol as a second choice.
    - Consider non-pharmacologic methods of pain control include local warming of abdomen and lower back and transcutaneous electrical nerve stimulation (TENS).

  - Management of UTI:

    - Treat UTI, if present, prior to endourologic stone removal.
    - Perform urgent decompression (percutaneous drainage or ureteral stenting) in patients with evidence of infection and obstructing stone or any signs of sepsis with obstructing stones.

  - Treat all uncomplicated cases of urolithiasis in pregnancy conservatively, unless there are clinical indications for intervention.
  - For ureteral stones:

- Active stone removal is indicated if there is low likelihood of spontaneous passage, persistent pain despite adequate pain medication, persistent obstruction, or renal insufficiency.
- If there are no indications for active stone removal, initial observation with periodic evaluation recommended for patients with newly diagnosed small ureteral stones (generally < 6 mm, but no exact cutoff known).
- Offer alpha blockers as medical expulsion therapy to adults with distal ureteral stones ≥ 5 but ≤ 10 mm.
- If active stone removal is needed, the choice of procedure depends on stone composition, location, size, available equipment, and patient preference.

    ❖ Ureteroscopy recommended for patient with mid- or distal ureteral stones who are not candidates for or failed medical expulsion therapy, suspected cysteine or uric acid ureteral stones, and for proximal and distal ureteral stones ≥ 10 mm.
    ❖ Shock wave lithotripsy (SWL) indicated if patient with mid- or distal ureteral stones declines ureterorenoscopy or can be option for proximal and distal stones < 10 mm.
    ❖ Use percutaneous antegrade removal as an alternative when SWL not indicated or has failed, and when upper urinary tract is not amenable to retrograde ureterorenoscopy.

o For renal stones:

- If there are no indications for active stone removal, consider observation for asymptomatic, stable renal stones.
- Indications for active stone removal include stone growth, stones in patients at high risk for stone formation, obstruction due to stones, infection, symptoms, large stone size, and patient preference.

- If active stone removal is needed, the choice of procedure depends on stone composition, location, size available equipment, and patient preference.

❖ For symptomatic calyceal diverticular stones, preferentially use endoscopic therapy (ureterorenoscopy, percutaneous nephrolithotomy, laparoscopic surgery, robotic surgery).
❖ For symptomatic non-lower pole renal stone burden ≤ 20 mm, offer SWL or ureterorenoscopy; if > 20 mm, offer percutaneous nephrolithotomy as first-line therapy.
❖ For stone in lower pole, management is typically SWL or endourology but choice also depends on size and presence of unfavorable factors for SWL.

   o For Steinstrasse, consider percutaneous nephrostomy if associated with UTI/fever or shock wave lithotripsy or ureteroscopy for large stone fragments.
   o Consider follow-up within 6 months of starting treatment with single 24-hour urine specimen for stone risk factors to assess response to dietary and/or medical therapy, and then at least annually.
   o To reduce recurrence risk:
      - Increase fluid intake spread through the day to achieve urine volume ≥ 2-2.5 L/day.
      - Consider criteria for high risk of recurrence to determine if secondary prevention is indicated.
      - Consider specific prevention strategies as guided by results of metabolic evaluation and stone composition analysis. For example:

- ❖ For calcium stones, consider pharmacologic monotherapy with thiazide diuretic, citrate, or allopurinol to prevent recurrent nephrolithiasis in patients with active disease in whom increased fluid intake fails to reduce the formation of stones.
- ❖ For struvite and infection stones, surgically remove stone material as completely as possible and prescribe antibiotics in patients with persistent bacteriuria.

Section 11: Neurology

Cerebrovascular Accident (CVA)

- Also known as stroke, is an episode of acute neurological dysfunction persisting > 24 hours with acute infarction or hemorrhage.
- Transient ischemic attack (TIA): occurs when blood flow to part of the brain stops for a short period of time, often less than 24 hours before disappearing. It can mimic stroke-like symptoms.

  o New definition for the TIA includes that impaired blood flow from 5 minutes to less than 1 hr.

- Strokes are generally classified into:

  o Ischemic stroke:

    ▪ Ischemic strokes (80% of stroke) are caused by large artery atherosclerosis (embolus or thrombosis), small vessel occlusion (lacunar), or cardioembolism (often from AFib).

  o Hemorrhagic stroke:

    ▪ Hemorrhagic strokes are typically due to intracerebral hemorrhage or subarachnoid hemorrhage. The most common mechanism of intracerebral hemorrhage is hypertensive small-vessel disease, causing small lipohyalinotic aneurysms that rupture.

- Risk factors for stroke include:

  o History of TIA, hypertension, myocardial infarction, atrial fibrillation, left atrial enlargement, smoking, heavy alcohol use, diabetes, obesity, high cholesterol, and carotid artery stenosis.

- Clinical features include:

    o Speech difficulty and hemiparesis.
    o Extremity or facial weakness, arm or leg numbness, confusion, headache, and dizziness.
    o Neurological exam may reveal focal weakness affecting the arm, leg, and/or face, aphasia or dysarthria, hemiparetic or ataxic gait, eye movement abnormalities, spatial neglect, and visual field defects.

- Diagnosis:

    o Initial assessment should include calculation of a formal stroke score, such as National Institutes of Health Stroke Scale (NIHSS), for diagnostic and prognostic classification of stroke severity.
    o Emergent studies to evaluate suspected acute stroke and differentiate stroke from other conditions including:

        ▪ Noncontrast head CT, is the best choice for diagnosing subarachnoid hemorrhage, absolute contraindication to thrombolytic therapy.
        ▪ Diffusion-weight brain MRI is more sensitive for diagnosing acute ischemic stroke.

    o Continuous cardiac monitoring is recommended for a minimum of 24 hours.
    o Other tests as indicated by the clinical presentation such as a pregnancy test, toxicology screen, blood alcohol level, arterial blood gas, chest radiography, lumbar puncture (to rule out CNS infection, or if a subarachnoid hemorrhage is suspected and there is no evidence of blood in subarachnoid space on neuroimaging), and electroencephalography.

- Management:

    o Admit patient to acute stroke unit care if available for neurologic and cardiac monitoring, as associated with decreased mortality.

- Thrombolytics (tissue-type plasminogen activator [t-PA], Activase) are recommended for patients with an acute ischemic stroke who have a measurable neurologic deficit if treatment can be started quickly enough and the patient has no contraindication.
- Contraindications vary across guidelines and drug marketing authorization but usually include:

  - Any evidence of intracranial hemorrhage on neuroimaging, or symptoms of subarachnoid hemorrhage.
  - Onset of symptoms greater than 3 to 4.5 hours prior to therapy, or unknown time of onset of symptoms.
  - Severe stroke, based on NIHSS score > 26 or ischemic signs involving > one-third of middle cerebral artery territory on neuroimaging.
  - Seizure at stroke onset.
  - Platelet count < 100,000/mm^3 or abnormal coagulation tests including INR > 1.7 or PT > 15 sec.
  - Blood glucose level < 50 mg/dL or > 400 mg/dL.
  - Recent procedure (in past 7 days) or surgery (in past 2 weeks or 3 months), or trauma.
  - History of recent bleeding, or comorbidities (e.g., HTN, DM, pericarditis, aneurysm…).

- Most guidelines recommend alteplase for carefully selected patients within 3 hours of acute ischemic stroke and also 3-4.5 hours after stroke onset.
- t-PA within 3 hours has evidence for improved functional outcomes but increases risk of intracranial hemorrhage within 7 days, and does not appear to affect mortality.
- Antihypertensives are generally not recommended in the setting of acute ischemic unless the systolic blood pressure is > 220 mmHg or the diastolic is > 120 mmHg.
- If patient has high BP but is otherwise eligible for t-PA, BP may be lowered to < 185/110 mmHg using medications such as IV Labetalol or IV Nicardipine infusion to meet eligibility criteria and then maintain BP < 180/105 mmHg for at least 24 hours after t-PA.

- Aspirin should be started 24-48 hours after an ischemic stroke in most patients to reduce the risk of death, dependency, and recurrent stroke.
- Early mobilization is recommended for less severely affected patients and early supported discharge is recommended for patients with a mild or moderate stroke.
- Decompressive surgery is recommended for:

    - Malignant edema of the cerebral hemispheres.
    - A space-occupying cerebellar infarction.

- All patients with stroke should have a formal swallowing evaluation prior to oral intake and should have reassessment throughout their hospital stay even if no dysphagia is seen on the initial evaluation.

- Complications following stroke include:

    - Persistent neurologic dysfunction.
    - Swallowing dysfunction, or taste disturbances.
    - Pneumonia.
    - Myocardial infarction.
    - Heart failure.
    - Cardiac arrhythmias.
    - Seizures, or delirium.
    - Post-stroke depression.
    - Venous thromboembolism.

- Interventions for primary prevention of stroke include:

    - Heart-healthy diet low in sodium.
    - Exercise.
    - Weight reduction.
    - Blood pressure control.
    - Smoking cessation.
    - Avoidance of heavy alcohol consumption
    - Statin, aspirin, or antithrombotic therapy when indicated.

- Secondary prevention of stroke relies heavily on risk factor reduction such as:

    o Increased physical activity.
    o Use of statins.
    o Blood pressure reduction.

Transient Ischemic Attack (TIA)

- TIA is a transient episode of neurologic dysfunction caused by focal ischemic of the brain, spinal cord, or retina without evidence of acute infarction on neuroimaging.
- Transient neurologic dysfunction with evidence of infarction on neuroimaging is referred to as transient symptoms with infarction (TSI).
- Causes:

  - TIAs may be caused by atheroemboli from carotid or vertebral artery stenosis, cardiogenic emboli in patients with valvular stenosis or arrhythmias such as atrial fibrillation, paradoxical emboli through intracardiac defects, aortic emboli, and in patients with hypercoagulable, prothrombotic, or hyperviscous states such as sickle cell disease, thrombocytosis, or leukemia.

- Risk Factors:

  - Metabolic conditions such as metabolic syndrome, type 2 DM, and chronic kidney disease.
  - Modifiable risk factors such as obesity, smoking, hyperlipidemia, heavy alcohol use, and substance abuse.
  - Cardiovascular conditions such as HTN, atrial fibrillation, carotid stenosis, or history of prior MI, nonischemic cardiomyopathies, TIA, or stroke.
  - Hormone replacement therapy and oral contraceptives.

- Clinical Features and Diagnosis:

  - Neurologic symptoms consistent with cerebral ischemia from the anterior circulation include:

- Motor or sensory dysfunction of the contralateral face and/or contralateral extremities.
- Ipsilateral vision loss or homonymous hemianopia.
- Speech disturbance such as aphasia or dysarthria.

o Neurologic symptoms consistent a posterior circulation event (vertebrobasilar circulation) may include:

- Motor or sensory dysfunction of the ipsilateral face and/or contralateral extremities (crossed pattern).
- Visual loss in one or both homonymous visual fields including cortical blindness and Anton syndrome (lack of awareness of blindness).
- Brainstem and cerebellar findings such as ataxia, vertigo, diplopia, dysphagia, and dysarthria.

o In patients referred for a suspected TIA or minor stroke, the most frequent noncerebrovascular diagnosis include migraine, syncope, seizure, psychiatric conditions, vertigo, and peripheral nerve conditions.

o Initial blood tests include (CBC for the evidence of polycythemia, Chemistry panel, Coagulation profile, Lipid profile, Fasting glucose, Cardiac markers including troponin).

o Neuroimaging with MRI or CT should be obtained within 24 hours of symptoms onset.

o An ECG should be obtained to assess for arrhythmia.

o Noninvasive vascular imaging is recommended for cervical and intracranial vessels with ultrasound, CT angiography, or MR angiography.

o Use a validated scoring system, such as the $ABCD^2$ score to calculate the risk:

- **A**ge ≥ 60 years (1 point).
- **B**lood pressure ≥ 140/90 mmHg (1 point).
- **C**linical features of the TIA:

❖ Unilateral weakness (2 points).
❖ Speech impairment (1 point).

- **D**uration of symptoms:

    ❖ 10-59 minutes (1 point).
    ❖ ≥ 60 minutes (2 points).

- **D**iabetes (1 point).

ABCD^2 Score	2-day Stroke Risk	Comment
0-3	1.0%	Hospital observation may be unnecessary without another indication (e.g., new atrial fibrillation)
4-5	4.1%	Hospital observation justified in most situations
6-7	8.1%	Hospital observation worthwhile

- Management:

    o Risk factor reduction through statin therapy, BP reduction, smoking cessation, and avoidance of heavy alcohol use should be implemented to prevent stroke.
    o Antiplatelet agents should be used rather than anticoagulation for patients with nonembolic TIA, such as:

- Clopidogrel 75 mg/day.
- A combination of aspirin 25 mg + extended release dipyridamole 200 mg BID.
- Aspirin 50-325 mg/day.

o Use oral anticoagulation in patients with atrial fibrillation.
o For patients with carotid artery stenosis:

- Perform carotid endarterectomy for patients with perioperative morbidity and mortality risk estimated < 6% (based on age, sex, comorbidities, and surgeon's success rate) and with ipsilateral severe (70%-99%) stenosis or moderate (50%-69%) stenosis.

Heatstroke

- It is defined as a body temperature higher than 41.1°C associated with neurologic dysfunction.
- Classifications:

  o There are 2 forms of heatstroke exist:

     - *Exertional heatstroke (EHS):* generally occurs in young individuals who engage in strenuous physical activity for a prolonged period of time in a hot environment.
     - *Classic non-exertional heatstroke (NEHS):* more commonly affects sedentary elderly individuals, persons who are chronically ill, and very young persons. It occurs during environmental heat waves and is more common in areas that do not typically experience periods of prolonged hot weather.

- Causes:

  o Increased heat production:

     - Can result from infections, sepsis, encephalitis, stimulant drugs (including cocaine and amphetamines), thyroid storm, drug withdrawal, physical exercise, convulsions.

  o Decreased heat loss:

     - Dermatological diseases, drugs (including barbiturates, beta-blockers, CCBs, diuretics, anticholinergic, neuroleptics, antihistamines), burns, high ambient temperatures.

- Reduced ability to acclimatize:
    - Persons at the extremes of age may be less able to generate adequate physiologic responses to heat stress. Diuretics use and hypokalemia can also impair accommodation to heat stress.
- Reduced behavioral responsiveness:
    - Infants, patients who are bedridden, and patients who are chronically ill are at risk for heatstroke because they are unable to control their environment and water intake.

- Clinical features:
    - Exertional heatstroke:
        - It is characterized by hyperthermia, diaphoresis, and an altered sensorium, which may manifest suddenly during extreme physical exertion in a hot environment.
        - A number of symptoms (e.g., abdominal and muscular cramping, nausea, vomiting, diarrhea, headache, dizziness, dyspnea, weakness) commonly precede the heatstroke and may remain unrecognized. Syncope and loss of consciousness also are observed commonly before the development of EHS.
    - Non-exertional heatstroke:
        - It is characterized by hyperthermia, anhidrosis, and an altered sensorium, which develop suddenly after a period of prolonged elevations in ambient temperatures (i.e., heat waves). Core body temperatures greater than 41°C are diagnostic, although heatstroke may occur with lower core body temperatures.

- Numerous CNS symptoms, ranging from minor irritability to delusions, irrational behavior, hallucinations, and coma have been described. Other possible CNS symptoms include seizures, cranial nerve abnormalities, cerebellar dysfunction, and opisthotonos.

    o Tachycardia to rates exceeding 130 beats per minute is common.
    o Examination of the eyes may reveal nystagmus and oculogyric episodes due to cerebellar injury.
    o Acute kidney injury is a common complication of heatstroke and may be due to hypovolemia, low cardiac output, and myoglobinuria (from rhabdomyolysis).

- Management:

    o Once heatstroke is suspected, cooling must begin immediately and must be continued during the patient's resuscitation. The American College of Sports Medicine recommends that cooling be initiated at the scene, before transporting the patient to an ED.
    o Apply ice packs to the patient's armpit, groin, neck, and back. Because these areas are rich with blood vessels close to the skin, cooling them may reduce body temperature.
    o Antipyretics (e.g., acetaminophen, aspirin, other NSAIDs) have no role in the treatment of heatstroke because antipyretics interrupt the change in the hypothalamic set point caused by pyrogens; they are not expected to work on a healthy hypothalamus that has been overloaded, as in the case of heatstroke.
    o Immediate administration of benzodiazepines is indicated in patients with agitation and shivering, to stop excessive production of heat.
    o Recommendations on the administration of IV fluids depends on the presence of hypovolemia.
    o Treatment of rhabdomyolysis involves infusion of large amounts of IV fluids up to 10 liters, alkalization of the urine, and infusion of mannitol.
        - Urine output should be maintained at 3 mL/kg/hour to minimize the risk of renal failure.

Headache

- Headache is defined as diffuse pain in various parts of the head, with the pain not confined to the area of distributing of a nerve.
- Headache is classified into:

  o *PRIMARY:*

    - Tension-type headache:

      ❖ It consists of bilateral head pain of mild-moderate intensity with a pressing or tightening quality. It may be described as a "band around the head".
      ❖ It can last 30 minutes to 7 days.
      ❖ Pericranial muscle tenderness on palpation is the most common abnormal finding on exam.
      ❖ Neuroimaging is indicated for patients who present with signs or symptoms suggesting increased risk of intracranial pathology.
      ❖ Simple analgesics and NSAIDs are the first-line options.
      ❖ First-line medication for prophylaxis is amitriptyline 30-75 mg/day.

    - Migraine headache:

      ❖ It is typically unilateral with a pulsating quality and may be preceded by a prodromal aura that consists of sensory, motor, or language symptoms.
      ❖ Classic aura occurs 5-20 minutes prior to the onset of headache and usually includes flashes (phosphenes), speaks, geometric forms, shimmering, or scotomata but

may also manifest as a wide variety of neurologic symptoms such as focal numbness or weakness.
- ❖ Headaches are classically unilateral, pulsating, have a gradual onset, and last 4-72 hours.
- ❖ Common triggers for headaches include menses, stress, exertion, sleep disturbance, odors, caffeine withdrawal, and dietary items such as cheese, wine, chocolate, monosodium glutamate (MSG), and hot dogs.
- ❖ Diagnose migraine in patients with a typical headache pattern after ≥ 5 attacks for migraine without aura and ≥ 2 attacks for migraine with aura.
- ❖ For treatment of migraine attack:

  - ➢ Acetaminophen 1 g or NSAIDs such as ibuprofen, naproxen, or aspirin are recommended first-line therapies for mild-to-moderate headaches and be taken at onset of aura or as soon as migraine onset is recognized.
  - ➢ Consider combination products such as acetaminophen/aspirin/caffeine combination (Excedrin Migraine) and acetaminophen/isometheptene/dichloralphenazone combination (Midrin) as effective first-line agents for mild-to-moderate migraine.
  - ➢ Consider antiemetics such as prochlorperazine (Compazine) and metoclopramide (Reglan) as adjunct treatment for migraine-associated nausea and vomiting, or as monotherapy by rectal, IM, or IV route for migraine pain in patients unable to take oral medication.
  - ➢ Migraine-specific agents recommended for moderate-to-severe migraine, or mild-to-moderate migraine that is not responsive to therapy include:
    - ⚜ Triptans 50-100 mg PO, SC, or intranasally.
    - ⚜ Dihydroergotamine (DHE) intranasally, can also be given IV, IM, or SC.

- ❖ Migraine prophylaxis strategies with strongest support for first-line use include propranolol (target dose 80-160 mg/day) or metoprolol (target dose 100-200 mg/day), and topiramate (target dose 50 twice daily).

- Cluster headache:

  - ❖ It is an uncommon primary headache disorder characterized by almost daily attacks of excruciating unilateral periorbital pain with ipsilateral cranial autonomic symptoms.
  - ❖ Attacks last 15 minutes to 3 hours and usually occur in bouts or clusters of weeks to months duration, with remission periods lasting 1-12 months.
  - ❖ Typical onset is between ages 10 and 39 years, and it is more common in men.
  - ❖ Patients usually present with excruciating unilateral headache characterized by sharp, piercing, throbbing, or burning periorbital pain. The pain usually at maximum intensity for duration of attack and then ending abruptly.
  - ❖ Ipsilateral cranial autonomic signs accompany headache in most patients and may include lacrimation, facial sweating, edema of face and eyelid, nasal congestion, rhinorrhea, and conjunctival injection.
  - ❖ Cluster headache needs to be distinguished from migraine headache and from trigeminal neuralgia.
  - ❖ First-line treatments to abort a cluster headache during an acute attack include:

    - ➢ 100% oxygen at ≥ 7 L/minute for ≥ 15 minutes via non-rebreathing face mask (flow rate of ≥ 10 L/minute or up to 15 L/minute may be needed).
    - ➢ Sumatriptan 6 mg SC injection.
    - ➢ Zolmitriptan 5 mg or 10 mg intranasal spray.

- ❖ For prophylaxis of episodic cluster headache during a cluster episode:

    - ➢ Use verapamil 80 mg PO TID with increase by 80 mg/dose every 2 weeks to maximum of 960 mg/day as first-line for prophylaxis of episodic cluster headache.
    - ➢ Patients treated with verapamil require ECG monitoring for heart block at baseline, before any change in dose, and 10 days following any dose change.

- o *SECONDARY:*

    - Acute narrow-angle glaucoma (unilateral, halos around lights, decreased visual acuity).
    - Encephalitis or (fever, altered mental status, seizures, focal neurological deficits).
    - Giant cell arteritis (age > 55 years, unilateral throbbing pain, pain when combing hair, visual disturbance, jaw claudication, fever, weight loss, sweats, temporal artery tenderness, proximal myalgias).
    - Idiopathic intracranial hypertension (migraine-like headache, diplopia, pulsatile tinnitus, loss of peripheral vision, papilledema).
    - Meningitis.
    - Subarachnoid hemorrhage (peak intensity a few seconds after headache onset "thunderclap headache", vomiting, syncope obtundation).
    - Subdural hematoma (chronic, sleepiness, altered mental status, hemiparesis, papilledema, presence of risk factors such as elderly, coagulopathy, dementia).

Multiple Sclerosis

- Multiple sclerosis (MS) is an inflammatory and neurodegenerative disease of the brain and spinal cord resulting in episodes of neurologic dysfunction that often recover (but the degree of recovery can vary and may have a gradually progressive course).
- Lesions are disseminated in time and space (with episodes affecting separate sites in the CNS, occurring at least 30 days apart).
- MS is an autoimmune disease likely due to a combination of genetic predisposition and environmental influence.
- The onset is usually before age 50 years and is more common in women.
- Clinical features include:

    o Spinal cord involvement (myelitis) with partial sensory or motor dysfunction, Lhermitte sign, or bowel and bladder dysfunction.
    o Brainstem involvement, potentially leading to vision difficulties, impaired swallowing and speech, vertigo, and pseudobulbar palsy.
    o Cerebrum involvement, which may result in cognitive impairment, depression, upper motor neuron signs, and unilateral motor or sensory deficits.
    o Cerebellar involvement causing problems with balance, vertigo, and/or impaired coordination.
    o Worsening of neurological symptoms with high body temperature (Uhthoff's phenomenon).

- Diagnosis:

    o 80% of patients will present initially with a clinically isolated syndrome before clinically definite MS is diagnosed.
    o Patients with suspected MS should be referred for a neurological consult.

- o Obtain MRI of the brain and spinal cord with and without contrast (although a diagnosis of MS should not be based on MRI findings alone).
- o The diagnosis of MS should be made using established current criteria (such as revised 2010 international diagnostic criteria) after:
    - Assessing that episodes are consistent with an inflammatory process.
    - Excluding alternative diagnoses.
    - Establishing that lesions have developed at different times and are in different anatomical locations for diagnosis of relapsing-remitting MS.
    - Establishing progressive neurological deterioration over > 1 year for diagnosis of primary progressive MS.

- Management:

  - o For clinically isolated syndrome (a neurologic presentation suggestive of MS), treatments to reduce progression to clinically definite MS include:
    - Interferon beta-1b.
    - Interferon beta-1a given either once weekly or 3 times weekly.
    - Glatiramer acetate.
    - IV immunoglobulin (IVIG).
    - Teriflunomide.

  - o For treatment of acute relapse:
    - Consider glucocorticoids in any patient with an acute attack of MS due to short-term benefit on the speed of functional recovery.
    - Glucocorticoids dosing options include oral methylprednisolone 500 mg/day for 5 days and IV methylprednisolone 1 g/day for 3-5 days.

- Plasmapheresis should be considered for adjunctive treatment of exacerbations of relapsing-remitting MS.

o For progressive MS, use of either interferon beta or glatiramer acetate is not recommended for patients with progressive, nonrelapsing forms of MS.

o Disease-modifying therapies for relapsing-remitting MS:

- Immunomodulatory drugs should be initiated at the time of diagnosis.
- Immunomodulatory options with evidence for efficacy include:
    - Interferon beta.
    - Glatiramer acetate.

o Treatment of selected specific impairments:

- For ambulation and mobility impairments, consider Dalfampridine, exercise therapy, or vestibular or multidisciplinary rehabilitation.
- For upper extremity tremor, consider botulinum toxin type A.
- For central neuropathic pain, consider gabapentin, pregabalin, amitriptyline, or duloxetine as 1st-line treatment. Second-line option is tramadol or opioids if used for short-term use. Consider cannabinoids for refractory pain.
- For urinary symptoms, consider oxybutynin or tolterodine and a bladder rehabilitation program. If refractory symptoms, consider bladder wall injection with botulinum toxin type A.

Table 1
Clinical Features that May Help Distinguish MS from Other Etiologies[6]

Clinical Features Suggestive of MS

- Onset between ages 15 and 50
- Involvement of multiple areas of the CNS (brain and spinal cord)
- Optic neuritis
- Lhermitte's sign
- Internuclear ophthalmoplegia
- Fatigue
- Worsening with elevated body temperature (Uhthoff's phenomenon)

Clinical Features NOT Suggestive of MS

- Onset before age 10 or after age 60
- Involvement of the peripheral nervous system
- Bilateral visual loss/visual field cut
- Rigidity, sustained dystonia
- Cortical deficits, such as aphasia, apraxia, alexia, and neglect
- Deficit developing within minutes
- Early dementia

2010 McDonald criteria for MS

Attacks	Lesions	Additional requirements for MS diagnosis
2 or more	2 or more	None
2 or more	1	Dissemination in space demonstrated by MRI or further attack
1	2	Dissemination in time demonstrated by MRI or further attack
1	1	Dissemination in space and time demonstrated by MRI or further attack
0 Insidious neurological progression suggestive of MS		1 year of disease progression and 2 of the following: • Positive brain MRI • Positive spinal cord MRI • Positive CSF

Febrile Seizure

- Also called febrile convulsion, is a seizure occurring in a child aged 6 months to 5 years with a temperature ≥ 38 degrees C and no CNS infection, metabolic disturbance, or history of afebrile seizure.
- Febrile seizures are most commonly due to infections but the precise mechanism is unknown.
- There is an increased risk of febrile seizures after certain immunizations (such as DTaP, IPV, Hib) but the absolute risk is very small.
- Classification:

  o Simple febrile seizure (most common type):
    - Generalized tonic-clonic activity with no focal component, duration < 15 minutes.
    - Occurs no more than once in 24 hours.
    - No previous neurologic problems (i.e., meningitis or encephalitis).

  o Complex febrile seizure:
    - Duration > 15 minutes, associated with focal component, recurrence within 24 hours.

- Diagnosis:

  o If simple febrile seizure, blood testing should be done only if it is useful for identifying source of fever, not as part of seizure evaluation.
  o Consider urinalysis and urine culture to identify UTI if it is clinically suspected as source of fever.

- Perform lumbar puncture in a child with febrile seizure and history or physical exam suggestive of meningitis or intracranial infection.
  - Neuroimaging and EEG are not recommended for the evaluation of simple febrile seizure in a neurologically healthy child (only for follow-up in children with complex or recurrence febrile seizures, or with neurologic abnormalities).

- Management:

  - Most simple febrile seizures will have stopped before presentation to a healthcare provider and will not require antiepileptic medication.
  - For febrile status epilepticus, a seizure lasting > 5 minutes, or repeated seizures:

    - Treat with lorazepam 0.1 mg/kg IV bolus; this may be repeated once after 5-10 minutes if needed (other options include IM midazolam, intranasal or rectal benzodiazepines).

  - For the prevention of febrile seizure recurrence:

    - Continuous or intermittent anticonvulsant therapy is not recommended for children with single or recurrent simple febrile seizure.
    - Antipyretic agents during fever may not reduce risk for recurrent febrile seizure.

Status Epilepticus

- Status epilepticus (SE) is a condition characterized by a prolonged period of either continuous seizure activity or recurrent seizure activity without a return to baseline.
- The condition results either from failure of mechanisms responsible for seizure termination or from initiation of mechanisms, which lead to abnormally prolonged seizures.
- International League Against Epilepsy (ILAE) criteria varies by seizure type:

    - ≥ 5 minutes for tonic clinic seizures.
    - ≥ 10 minutes for focal seizures without impaired consciousness.
    - $\geq 10\text{-}15$ minutes for absence seizures.

- Neurocritical Care Society (NCS) criteria is ≥ 5 minutes of either continuous clinical or electrographic seizure activity, or recurrent seizure activity without return to baseline between seizures.
- Etiology:

    - Common causes in children include febrile seizure, central nervous system infection, inborn error of metabolism, and ingestion.

- Diagnosis:

    - Diagnostic workup should be completed as soon as possible and occur simultaneously and in parallel with treatment.
    - Immediate testing should include:

        - Fingerstick glucose.
        - Vital signs (including oxygen saturation).

- Blood tests, including glucose, CBC, basic metabolic panel, calcium, magnesium.

  o Consider additional testing based on clinical presentation, including:

  - Electroencephalogram.
  - Neuroimaging with CT or MRI should be obtained in a patient without a known seizure disorder.
  - Lumbar puncture.
  - Toxicology screen (urine and blood).

- Management:

  o Stabilization and monitoring should be started immediately and continued in parallel with pharmacologic treatment, including:

  - Assessing and supporting airway, breathing, circulation.
  - Performing neurologic examination.
  - Obtaining IV access and diagnostic tests.

  o The goal of pharmacologic treatment is rapid cessation of seizure activity.
  o Give benzodiazepines as the first-line treatment for SE, preferred options include:

  - Lorazepam 0.1 mg/kg IV, may repeat dose once.
  - Midazolam 5 mg IM if 13-40 kg, 10 mg IM if > 40 kg, or 0.2 mg/kg IM.
  - Diazepam 0.15-0.2 mg/kg IV, may repeat dose once.

  o If IV or IM formulations are not feasible or available, consider:

  - Buccal intranasal midazolam 0.5 mg/kg buccally, 0.2 mg/kg intranasally.
  - Rectal diazepam 0.2-0.5 mg/kg per rectum.

- Second-line options for benzodiazepine-refractory SE include the following:

    - Valporic acid 20-40 mg/kg IV.
    - Fosphenytoin 20 mg/kg phenytoin equivalent IV.
    - Levetiracetam 20-60 mg/kg IV.
    - Phenobarbital 15-20 mg/kg IV.

- For refractory SE, a continuous infusion of an antiepileptic drug should be started and titrated until there is cessation of electrographic seizures or burst suppression.

    - Midazolam, thiopental, propofol (contraindicated in children), and pentobarbital are the agents recommended for refractory SE with all except midazolam requiring mechanical ventilation due to medication-induced respiratory depression.

- In children with SE refractory to pharmacologic treatments, options that may be considered include:

    - Ketogenic diet.
    - Therapeutic hypothermia.
    - Immunomodulation.
    - Neurosurgery.
    - Vagal stimulation.
    - Electroconvulsive therapy.

Bell's Palsy

- Bell palsy is a subacute weakness of the facial nerve (the 7th cranial nerve).
- It may be partial or complete palsy.
- It may be idiopathic or secondary to infections such as Lyme disease or herpes infections.
- Risk factors DM and URTI.
- Evaluation:

    o Diagnosis is made clinically.
    o Patients typically present with acute onset of unilateral facial weakness, which may result in asymptomatic smile or trouble fully closing eyelids, hyperacusis (sensitivity to sound), or unilateral loss of taste sensation.
    o No testing is typically needed but consider testing for Lyme disease (erythema migrans).
    o External ear canal should always be checked for presence of vesicles consistent with Ramsay-Hunt syndrome.

Grade	Description
Grade 1	Normal facial function in all areas
Grade 2	Mild dysfunction, slight weakness only seen in close inspection, complete closure of eye
Grade 3	Moderate dysfunction, obvious weakness, eye closure is complete with max. effort
Grade 4	Facial weakness is obvious and disfiguring, eye closure incomplete
Grade 5	Severe dysfunction, minimal movement, eye closure incomplete, slight mouth movement
Grade 6	Total paralysis, no movement, loss of tone, no synkinesia, contracture, of hemifacial spasm

- Management:

    - Recommend eye protection if the patient cannot fully close the eye, which may include lubrication (eyedrops or ointment) and eyelid taping.
    - Offer corticosteroids to patients with new-onset (usually < 72 hours) disease to increase the likelihood of full recovery.

        - Prednisone 25 mg twice daily for 10 days.
        - Prednisolone 60 mg orally once daily for 5 days, then tapered by 10 mg each day until day 10.
        - Prednisolone 1 mg/kg/day for 10 days in children (ONLY use in children if complete).

    - Antiviral therapy (such as acyclovir) should not be offered as sole therapy, but may be considered in conjunction with corticosteroids.

Consider adding facial exercise therapy to pharmacologic therapy to improve functional outcomes

Benign Paroxysmal Positional Vertigo (BPPV)

- BPPV is an inner ear disorder manifested by repeated episodes of spinning sensation triggered by changes in head position relative to gravity.
- BPPV results from a small crystal of calcium carbonate (otoconia) entering a semicircular canal, usually affecting the posterior canal but it can also affect the horizontal or anterior semicircular canals.
- Most cases are idiopathic, but known causes of BPPV include head trauma, ear surgery, and inner ear disorders.
- Prognosis is excellent, as most patients with idiopathic BPPV experience resolution of symptoms within days or weeks. Recurrence is common.
- Evaluation:

    o Suspect BPPV in patients with a history and physical exam consistent with repeated brief (seconds) episodes of vertigo immediately following changes in head position and without signs or symptoms of hearing loss or an underlying neurological disorder.
    o Assess patients with BPPV for factors that modify management, including impaired mobility or balance, CNS disorders, lack of home support, and/or increased risk of falling.
    o Confirm posterior (and rarely anterior) canal BPPV using the Dix-Hallpike maneuver.

      - There is a latency period of about 5-20 seconds between completion pf the Dix-Hallpike maneuver and onset of nystagmus and vertigo.
      - Nystagmus is typically torsional; a subset of patients may also have an upward (posterior canal) or rarely, downward (anterior canal) beating component.

- Initial vertigo increases and then resolves within 60 seconds from onset of nystagmus.
- After the patient sits up, the nystagmus recurs but in the opposite direction.
- Test is positive for downward ear.

- If the history is suggestive of BPPV in a patient with a negative Dix-Hallpike maneuver, perform the supine roll test to assess for horizontal canal BPPV.
- Differentiate BPPV from the other most common causes of vertigo, acute vestibular neuronitis and Meniere disease, and from other causes of positional vertigo such as postural hypotension, central positional vertigo, and vestibular migraine.
- Absence of nystagmus accompanying vertigo during the Dix-Hallpike maneuver in a patient with otherwise suggestive history does not rule out BPPV.
- Do not perform radiographic imaging and vestibular testing unless diagnosis is uncertain or there are other signs or symptoms unrelated to BPPV.

- Management:

  - Educate patients about the impact of BPPV on their safety, potential for disease recurrence, and importance of follow-up.
  - Treat, or refer to a clinician who can treat, patients with posterior or anterior canal BPPV or subjective BPPV using a particle (canalith) repositioning maneuver, such as Epley maneuver or Semont maneuver. The affected ear in posterior canal BPPV is the ear that was positive on Dix-Hallpike testing.

    - Perform the modified Epley maneuver on patients of all ages.
    - Self-treatment with any of the above canalith repositioning maneuvers at home is an option.
    - Don't use post-procedure postural restrictions in patients treated with canalith repositioning procedure.

- Treat patients with horizontal canal BPPV with procedures such as the Gufoni maneuver, barbecue rotation, or head-shaking maneuver. Determining the affected ear can be complex and may require specialty referral after the initial diagnosis.
- BPPV should not be routinely treated with vestibular suppressant medications such as antihistamines and/or benzodiazepines.
- Reassess patients within 1 month after the initial period of observation or treatment to document resolution or persistent of symptoms.

Cervical Dystonia

- It is a movement disorder characterized by involuntary movement (twisting or repetitive) or abnormal posturing of the neck (head tilt and rotation) due to sustained or intermittent muscle contractions.
- It may be idiopathic, genetic, or secondary to multiple different factors such as brain injury (e.g. dystonic cerebral palsy, head trauma), exposure to drugs (e.g. Antidepressants, Antipsychotics, Dopamine agonists, Anticonvulsants) or toxins, vascular injuries (e.g. ischemia, hemorrhage, aneurysm), or tumors (e.g. brain tumor or paraneoplastic encephalitis).
- Patients often present with abnormal head and neck posture or movements (often repetitive).
- Tremor is common in patients with cervical dystonia.
- Voluntary action can often trigger or worsen dystonia, and dystonia may lessen when body is at rest. Dystonia usually disappears during sleep.
- The diagnosis is made clinically.
- Management:

    o Neuromuscular blocker such as *Botulinum toxin* type A (or type B if resistant to type A) is the first-line treatment for cervical dystonia.
    o Physical therapy.
    o Treating the secondary cause may help in relieving dystonia.
    o For patients with dopa-responsive dystonia, start chronic treatment with Levodopa after positive diagnostic trial, then adjust based on clinical response.

Section 12: Obstetrics and Gynecology

Antenatal Care

- Antenatal care (ANC) can be defined as the care provided by skilled health-care professionals to pregnant women and adolescent girls in order to ensure the best health conditions for both mother and baby during pregnancy.
- Goals of ANC:

  o ANC reduces maternal and perinatal morbidity and mortality both directly, through detection and treatment of pregnancy-related complications, and indirectly, through the identification of women and girls at increased risk of developing complications during labor and delivery, thus ensuring referral to an appropriate level of care.
  o In addition, as indirect causes of maternal morbidity and mortality such as HIV and malaria infections, contribute to approximately 25% of maternal deaths and near-misses, ANC also provides an important opportunity to prevent and manage concurrent diseases through integrated service delivery.

- Nutritional interventions recommendations:

  o Counseling about healthy eating and keeping physically active during pregnancy is recommended.
  o Daily oral iron and folic acid supplementation with 30 mg to 60 mg of elemental iron and 0.4 mg of folic acid (or 120 mg of elemental iron and 2.8 mg of folic acid once weekly) is recommended for pregnant women to prevent maternal anemia, puerperal sepsis, low birth weight, and preterm birth.

    - *60 mg of elemental iron = 300 mg of ferrous sulfate.*

- - In populations with low dietary calcium intake, daily calcium supplementation (1.5-2.0 g oral elemental calcium) is recommended to reduce the risk of preeclampsia.

- Maternal assessment:

  - Full blood count testing is the recommended method for diagnosing anemia in pregnancy.
  - Midstream urine culture is the recommended method for diagnosing asymptomatic bacteriuria (ASB) in pregnancy.
  - Hyperglycemia first detected at any time during pregnancy should be classified as either GDM or diabetes mellitus in pregnancy.
  - Health-care providers should ask all pregnant women about their tobacco use, alcohol and other substances (past and present).
  - HIV and syphilis testing is recommended to eliminate mother-to-child transmission.

- Fetal assessment:

  - One US scan before 24 weeks of gestation (early US) is recommended to estimate gestational age, improve detection of fetal anomalies and multiple pregnancies, and reduce induction of labor for post-term pregnancy.

- Preventive measure:

  - A seven-day antibiotic regimen is recommended for all pregnant women with ASB to prevent persistent bacteriuria, preterm birth and low birth weight.
  - Antenatal prophylaxis with anti-D immunoglobulin in non-sensitized Rh-negative pregnant women at 28 and 34 weeks of gestation to prevent RhD alloimmunization is recommended.
  - Tetanus toxoid vaccination is recommended for all pregnant women, depending on previous tetanus vaccination exposure, to prevent neonatal mortality from tetanus.

- Interventions for common physiologic symptoms:

    o Ginger, chamomile, vitamin B6 and/or acupuncture are recommended for the relief of nausea and vomiting in early pregnancy.
    o Advice on diet and lifestyle is recommended to prevent and relief heartburn in pregnancy. Antacid preparations can be offered as well.
    o Magnesium, calcium or non-pharmacological treatment options can be used for the relief of leg cramps in pregnancy.
    o Regular exercise throughout pregnancy is recommended to prevent low back and pelvic pain.
    o Wheat bran or other fiber supplements can be used to relieve constipation in pregnancy if the condition fails to respond to dietary modifications.
    o Non-pharmacological options, such as compression stockings, leg elevation and water immersion, can be used for the management of varicose veins and edema in pregnancy.

- WHO FANC model vs 2016 WHO ANC model:

    o The 2016 WHO ANC model replaces the previous four-visit focused ANC (FANC) model. within this model, the word "contact" has been used instead of "visit", as it implies an active connection between a pregnant woman and a health-care provider.

Infertility

- Infertility is defined as the inability to conceive after 1 year of unprotected sexual intercourse.
- *Male Infertility:*

    o The cause of infertility involves male factors alone in 30% of infertile couples.

    o The most common risk factors for male factor infertility is a history of cryptorchidism; other risk factors include:

    - DNA damage.
    - Endocrine pathology, such as hyperprolactinemia.
    - Exogenous administration of androgenic steroids.
    - Genetic conditions.
    - Genital tract obstruction due to congenital abnormalities, infection, or postsurgical complications.
    - Gonadotoxins.
    - Infections, including sexually transmitted diseases.
    - Obesity.
    - Testicular failure (primary and secondary).

    o Evaluation:

    - Initiate evaluation for male factor infertility in infertile couples who have not had pregnancy after 12 months of unprotected intercourse (or 6 months if female > 35 years old), or earlier if history and physical findings suggest specific infertility risk factors.
    - A complete history and physical should include (length of time trying to conceive, timing of intercourse, status of partner's workup, ejaculatory problems, prior infections, use

of lubricants, examination of patient for presence of secondary sexual characteristics and genital exam that looks for the presence of an absent or atrophic testicle and proximal hypospadias).
- Obtain a semen analysis as part of the initial evaluation. Repeat the semen analysis for confirmation if the first semen analysis shows abnormal results.
- Consider a postejaculatory urinalysis to detect sperm in men with ejaculate volume < 1 mL to exclude retrograde ejaculation.
- Offer cystic fibrosis transmembrane conductance regulator (CFTR) gene mutation testing to men with absence of 1 or both vas deferens on physical exam.
- Offer karyotype testing and Y chromosome microdeletion testing to men with unobstructive azoospermia or unexplained infertility and severe oligospermia (< 5-10 million/mL).

o Management:

- Encourage lifestyle changes such as avoiding tobacco and/or marijuana, reducing alcohol exposure, exercise and weight loss if obese, avoiding lubricants that may alter sperm, and avoiding increased scrotal temperature.
- Consider antioxidant supplementation in couples with male factor or unexplained fertility.
- For men with hypogonadotropic hypogonadism (offer gonadotropins "HCG 1500-3000 units subcutaneously and FSH 37.5-74 units IM 3 times/week" for improving fertility).
- Discontinue testosterone during treatment for infertility. Testosterone may be restarted after pregnancy is achieved.
- For men with hyperprolactinemia, use cabergoline as the first-line treatment.
- Do not offer varicocele repair if there is a normal semen analysis.

- Offer sperm retrieval via testicular sperm extraction if there is nonobstructive azoospermia, or via extraction or epididymal aspiration if there is obstructive azoospermia.

- *Female Infertility:*

  o Cause of infertility in couples may be multifactorial and may include:

    - Combined male and female factors in about 40%.
    - Ovulation disorders in about 21%-25%.
    - Tubal factors in about 14%-20%.
    - Cervical, uterine, or peritoneal disorders in about 10-13%.
    - Idiopathic (no identified male or female causes) in about 25-28%.

  o Evaluation:

    - History of dysfunctional bleeding and/or oligo/amenorrhea typically indicates ovulatory dysfunction.
    - Endocrine evaluation and/or imaging may be indicated in women with inconclusive results on history and physical.
    - Hysterosalpingography (HSG) may help detect suspected tubal and/or uterine abnormalities.
    - Hysteroscopy is the definitive method for diagnosis and treatment of intrauterine pathology, and is typically reserved for women with risk factors for tubal obstruction, such as endometriosis, previous pelvic infections, or ectopic pregnancy or intrauterine abnormalities detected by HSG.
    - Laparoscopy and chromotubation (with dilute solution or methylene blue or indigo carmine inserted via the cervix) may help detect tubal patency or proximal/distal tubal occlusive disease.

- Management:

    - Ovulation disorders:

        - Women with ovulation disorders due to hyperprolactinemia may benefit from dopamine agonists.

    - In women with mild tubal disease, tubal microsurgery or laparoscopic tubal surgery may help open tubes, although in vitro fertilization (IVF) may be a reasonable alternative given the increased risk of ectopic pregnancy.
    - In women with uterine disorders, surgical interventions may be beneficial.
    - In women with endometriosis-associated infertility, options include surgery or assisted reproductive technology, which may include pretreatment with hormonal therapies such as gonadotropin-releasing hormone agonists.
    - Intrauterine insemination (IUI) (with or without ovarian stimulation) may be considered for patients with social, cultural, or religious objections to IVF.

Menopause

- Menopause is a physiologic event characterized by loss of ovarian activity and permanent cessation of menses, diagnosed after 12 consecutive months of amenorrhea.
- This process occurs naturally, but can also be induced by medications, gynecologic surgery, chemotherapy, or radiation, often with sudden onset of symptoms in these circumstances.
- The mean age of onset of natural menopause is 51 years, with perimenopausal (transitional) symptoms often seen in women aged 40-58 years.
- Etiology:

    o Physiological: average age 51 years (follicular atresia).
    o Premature ovarian failure: before age 40 years (autoimmune disorder, infection, Turner's syndrome).
    o Iatrogenic: (surgical, radiation, chemotherapy).

- Clinical features include:

    o Vasomotor symptoms (hot flushes) > 50% of perimenopausal women.

        - Occurrence of vasomotor symptoms peaks about 1 year after the final menstrual period, with symptoms lasting an average of 4-10 years.
        - Symptoms spontaneously cease within 5 years of onset for most women.

    o Night sweats.
    o Insomnia.
    o Vaginal atrophy.

- o Sexual dysfunction.

- Diagnosis:

  - o Testing beyond history and physical is not typically needed for diagnosis but may help identify the stage of menopausal transition.
  - o Estradiol levels (form of the hormone estrogen) appear stable in early perimenopausal women.

    - Estradiol levels < 20 pg/mL may indicate menopause.

  - o FSH appears to have limited reliability for determining the start of perimenopause in women.

    - FSH levels > 30-40 milliunits/mL may indicate menopause.

  - o Vaginal pH > 4.5 may indicate perimenopause or menopause.

- Management:

  - o Lifestyle modifications may help reduce menopausal symptoms, including dietary calcium and vitamin D supplements, Black Cohesh, exercise, mind-body therapies.
  - o Vasomotor symptoms of menopause may improve with environmental modifications, hormonal therapies (systemic or local), and non-hormonal therapies.

    - Environmental modifications include layering of clothing, maintaining a lower ambient temperature, and consumption of cool drinks may help improve vasomotor symptoms associated with menopause.
    - Hormonal therapy with estrogen alone or in combination with progestin (for women with intact uterus) is the most effective treatment for vasomotor symptoms:

- ❖ Low-dose and ultra-low-dose estrogen therapy is associated with fewer adverse effects than higher doses.
- ❖ Transdermal or transvaginal estrogen should be considered for vasomotor symptom relief in women with hypertension, hypercholesterolemia, or at increased risk of cholelithiasis.

- Non-hormonal therapies for alleviation of vasomotor symptoms include SSRIs, SNRIs, clonidine, and gabapentin.
  - ❖ Paroxetine 7.5 mg/day is the only approved non-hormonal therapy for treatment of menopause-related vasomotor symptoms.

o Urogenital symptoms may be treated with hormonal and non-hormonal therapies:

- Local estrogen therapy is recommended to alleviate symptoms associated with vaginal atrophy in women without concurrent vasomotor symptoms.
- Systemic estrogen therapy is recommended for women with concurrent vasomotor and urogenital symptoms.
- Nonestrogen water-based or silicone-based vaginal lubricants and moisturizers may alleviate vaginal symptoms.

o Routine discontinuation of systemic estrogen at age 65 years is not recommended, as some women aged > 65 years may require continued systemic therapy.

o There are 3 types of hormone replacement therapy (HRT):

- Cyclical combined HRT (continuous estrogen, 12/28 days of progestogens; they cause regular withdrawal bleeds).
- Continuous combined HRT (continuous estrogen and progestogens; they can only be used 12 months after the last menstrual period).

- Estrogen only (continuous estrogen, they can only be used if the woman has had a hysterectomy).

o Side effects of HRT include:

- Abnormal uterine bleeding.
- Mastodynia (breast tenderness).
- Edema.
- Bloating.
- Heartburn.
- Nausea.
- Mood changes (especially in progesterone).

o Contraindications to HRT:

- Absolute contraindication:
  - ❖ Acute liver disease.
  - ❖ Undiagnosed vaginal bleeding.
  - ❖ Known or suspected uterine cancer/breast cancer.
  - ❖ Acute vascular thrombosis.
  - ❖ Cardiovascular disease.

- Relative contraindication:
  - ❖ Pre-existing uncontrolled HTN.
  - ❖ Uterine fibroids and endometriosis.
  - ❖ Familial hyperlipidemias.
  - ❖ Migraine headache.
  - ❖ Family history of estrogen-dependent cancer.
  - ❖ DM (with vascular disease).
  - ❖ Fibrocystic disease of the breasts.

Abnormal Uterine Bleeding (AUB)

- Abnormal uterine bleeding (AUB) describes a wide range of irregular bleeding patterns including acute or chronic heavy menstrual bleeding, abnormal duration of menstrual bleeding, as well as irregularities of menstrual cycle timing.
- Definitions:

    - *Polymenorrhea*: regular cycle interval < 24 days.
    - *Oligomenorrhea*: regular cycle interval > 40 days.
    - *Menorrhagia*: regular blood loss > 80 mL or menses > 7 days.
    - *Metrorrhagia*: irregular bleeding.
    - *Menometrorrhagia*: heavy and irregular bleeding.

- About 9-14% of reproductive-aged women are reported to have abnormal uterine bleeding.
- Causes include:

    - Structural abnormalities, such as endometrial polyps, uterine fibroids, adenomyosis, or malignancies.
    - Coagulopathies or bleeding disorders.
    - Ovulatory dysfunction.
    - Iatrogenic sources, such as medications, smoking, or breakthrough bleeding with use of intrauterine device or noncompliance with hormonal contraceptives.
    - Chlamydia genital infection.
    - Physical or psychological stress, or eating disorder.

- Evaluation:
    - Initial evaluation of women presenting with AUB should include details of bleeding pattern to help determine underlying etiology, physical exam, and pregnancy test.

- CBC is recommended if history of excessive blood loss.
- Additional testing is guided by patient history and response to treatment, and may include TSH, coagulation studies, endometrial biopsy, or further evaluation with US, saline infusion sonography, and/or hysteroscopy for persistent bleeding.

- Management:

  - Treatment for acute severe bleeding:

    - For women WITHOUT known or suspected bleeding disorder:
      - First-line treatment is a hormonal medication such as conjugated equine estrogen 25 mg IV every 4-6 hours for 24 hours or monophasic combined oral contraceptives with ethinyl estradiol 35 mcg TID for 7 days.
      - Consider antifibrinolytic drugs, such as tranexamic acid, in women with contraindications to hormonal medications.

    - For women with a known or suspected bleeding disorder:
      - Additional specific factor replacement may be required.
      - Intrauterine (endometrial) balloon tamponade is recommended with hormonal or hemostatic therapy for continued bleeding.

    - For women with hemodynamic instability or continued bleeding, consider intrauterine (endometrial) tamponade (Foley bulb), dilation and curettage, endometrial ablation, uterine artery embolization, or hysterectomy.

  - Treatment for women with anovulatory bleeding:

- Medical management is recommended for anovulatory bleeding due to an endocrinologic abnormality.
- Treatment regimens may include:

  ❖ Insertion of Levonorgestrel intrauterine device (Mirena).
  ❖ Combined oral contraceptives with ethinyl estradiol ≤ 35 mcg.
  ❖ Medroxyprogesterone acetate (Provera) 10 mg/day for 10-14 days per month.
  ❖ Metformin and other insulin-sensitizing drugs for irregular bleeding in women with polycystic ovary syndrome.

o Treatment of women with abnormal ovulatory bleeding and normal results on imaging may include:

- Medroxyprogesterone acetate 10 mg 21 days per month for 3-6 months.
- Insertion of Levonorgestrel intrauterine device.
- Trial of NSAIDs beginning first day of menses and continuing until menses cease.
- Tranexamic acid (Lysteda) 2 tablets (650 mg each) orally TID on days 1-5 of cycle.

o If excessive bleeding continues after a 3-6 months trial of pharmacological therapy, consider endometrial biopsy or referral for possible hysteroscopy, endometrial ablation, or hysterectomy.

Surgery may be indicated for anovulatory uterine bleeding in women with atypia or malignancy or abnormal bleeding due to structural malformations.

Antepartum Hemorrhage (APH)

- APH is any vaginal bleeding happens after 20 weeks of gestation.
- It is a medical EMERGENCY.
- Causes include:

    o Placenta previa, Abruptio placenta, Cervical causes (such as ectropion, trauma, polyps, and infection), and Uterine rupture.

- Placenta previa:

    o It defined as Lower uterine segment placenta (5 cm from the internal os or below the reflection of visceral peritoneum).
    o Grades:

    - Low implantation.
    - Reaches the internal os.
    - Partial, asymmetric.
    - Complete, central.

    o Risk factors: Multiparous, > 40 years, previous C-Section, IVF, smoking, previous placenta previa.
    o Associated with placenta accrete (endometrial invasion in 78%), placenta increta (myometrial invasion in 17%), and placenta percreta (serosa invasion in 5%).
    o Associated with IUGR, fetal abnormality, abruption placenta in 10% of the cases.
    o Clinical presentation: Painless bleeding, soft uterus, normal fetal heart, high presenting part, and malpresentation.
    o Vaginal exam is contraindicated!
    o Diagnosis: Clinical presentation then trans-vaginal ultrasound. MRI or OR (if in doubt).

- Complications: Shock, preterm labor, IUGR, malpresentation, IUFD, PROM, post-partum hemorrhage.
- Management:

    - For every patient: Admit, ABC, vital signs, hydration, fetal and maternal monitoring, labs (CBC, type and cross), Anti-D.
    - Consider vaginal delivery if the placenta is 4.5 cm from the internal os and absence of bleeding.
    - C-Section: grade 3 or 4, bleeding, within 2 cm from the internal os.
    - Mild bleeding:

        - <36 weeks → conservative
        - >36 weeks → C-Section

    - Moderate bleeding:

        - <34 weeks → resuscitation + steroid (conservative)
        - >34 weeks → C-Section

    - Severe bleeding: resuscitation then C-Section.

- Abruptio placenta:

  - It is defined as premature separation of the placenta.
  - External abruption (painful bleeding) Vs. Concealed (pain without bleeding).
  - Risk factors: Trauma, extreme of age, HTN and PET, PROM, smoking, thrombophilia, chorioamnionitis, previous abruption placenta, multiple pregnancy.
  - Diagnosis: Clinical (pain, bleeding, shock, hard and tender uterus. Ultrasound is used for (viability, AFI, Doppler, growth, and to exclude placenta previa).
  - Complications: Preterm labor, acute renal failure, DIC, uterine atony (Couvelaire uterus).

- o Management:

    - For every patient: Admit, ABC, vital signs, hydration, fetal and maternal monitoring, labs (CBC, type and cross), Anti-D.
    - 50% of the cases present at labor.
    - Conservative: <34 weeks, well baby and mother, mild bleeding.
    - Consider vaginal delivery low gestational age, dead baby, fully dilated cervix.
    - C-Section: distressed baby, severe bleeding.

- Uterine rupture:

    - o The most common cause of maternal morbidity.
    - o Clinical Features: Characterized by severe pain then it disappears, loss of station, floating fetus, absence or decreased fetal heart rate, fetal or maternal shock.
    - o Risk factors: previous c-section, multiple gestation, induction of labor, trauma, shoulder dystocia, forceps delivery.
    - o Management: Emergency laparotomy.

- Vasa previa:

    - o Clinical Feature: Onset of bleeding at rupture of membrane.
    - o Risk factors: bilobed placenta, succenturiate placenta, velamentous insertion of the cord.
    - o Diagnosis: Clinical, Ultrasound (Doppler).
    - o Management: Elective c-section after establishing the diagnosis before labor.

Postpartum Hemorrhage (PPH)

- Postpartum hemorrhage (PPH) describes abnormal or excessive blood loss that occurs after childbirth, generally in excess of 500 mL.
- Postpartum hemorrhage remains the leading cause of maternal death worldwide, and is the most common form of major obstetric hemorrhage.
- Risk factors for PPH include previous PPH, multiple gestation, placenta previa, fetal macrosomia, polyhydramnios, abnormal labor, high parity, previous uterine surgery (including C-section), clotting disorder, and therapeutic anticoagulation.
- Causes:

    o Tone (Uterine atony):

    - It is the most common cause of PPH (80-90%).
    - It occurs within first 24 hours.
    - *It occurs due to:*

        ❖ Labor (prolonged, precipitous, induced, augmented).
        ❖ Uterus (infection, over-distension).
        ❖ Placenta (abruption, previa).
        ❖ Maternal factors (grand multiparity, gestational HTN).
        ❖ Medications (MgSO4, β-adrenergic agonists, Halothane anesthesia).

    o Tissue:

    - Retained placenta "5%" (placenta undelivered after 30 min postpartum, it can result from abnormal placental implantation).
    - Retained blood clots in an atonic uterus.

- Gestational trophoblastic neoplasia.

o Trauma:

- Laceration (vagina, cervix, uterus), is the second most common (15%).
- Episiotomy.
- Hematoma (vaginal, vulvar, retroperitoneal).
- Uterine rupture (tearing of the uterus occurs most commonly in association with a previous scar on the uterus, typically Cesarean section).
- Uterine inversion (inversion of the uterus through cervix, it can result from excess cord traction with fundal placenta, or excessive use of tocolytics).

o Thrombin (Coagulopathy):

- It most identified prior to delivery (low platelet increases risk).
- Includes hemophilia, DIC, Aspirin use, ITP, TTP, vWD (most common).

- Evaluation:

o Clinical diagnosis is sufficient based on excessive blood loss after delivery, especially if signs or symptoms of hemodynamic instability are present.

- American College of Obstetrics and Gynecologists (ACOG) defines excessive blood loss as blood loss ≥ 1,000 mL regardless of route of delivery.
- Other criteria traditionally used include:
  ❖ Blood loss > 500 mL after vaginal delivery.
  ❖ Blood loss > 1,000 mL after cesarean delivery.

- o Blood tests including blood type and cross match, CBC, and coagulation studies should be obtained and repeated as clinically indicated.
- o Frequent monitoring of vital signs for hemodynamic instability and hypovolemic shock, and ongoing monitoring of fluid replacement, and use of blood products may be necessary to maintain hemodynamic stability.

- **Management:**

  - o Promptly establish IV access with ≥ 14-gauge peripheral IV for all patients with signs of PPH, and begin full resuscitative measures for postpartum patients with estimated blood loss > 1,000 ml and continued bleeding, or any signs of shock.
  - o Identify and treat the source of bleeding: one or more of "the 4 Ts" (tone, tissue, trauma, or thrombin) are often the cause of PPH.
  - o Consider tranexamic acid for management of PPH, particularly when initial medical therapy fails.
  - o Give 1 g (100 mg/mL) IV infusion at 1 mL per minute within 3 hours of birth in addition to standard care for clinically diagnosed PPH following vaginal birth or cesarean section.
  - o For PPH due to uterine atony:

    - Perform bimanual uterine massage.
    - Give uterotonic agents immediately.

      - ❖ Uterotonic agent of choice is oxytocin (Pitocin) 10-40 units IV in 0.5-1 L normal saline as continuous infusion or 10 units IM. Avoid undiluted rapid IV infusion as this may cause hypotension.
      - ❖ If oxytocin is not available or if bleeding is refractory to oxytocin, alternative uterotonics to consider include:

        - ✓ Ergot alkaloids, such as methylergonovine (Methergine) 0.2 mg IM every 2-4 hours, or

- ergonovine (ergometrine) 0.2-0.5 mg IM or slow-IV every 2 hours, or
- ✓ Misoprostol (Cytotec) which can be given orally, sublingually, or rectally.
- ✓ 15-methyl PGF (Carboprost, Hemabate) 0.25 mg IM or intramyometrially every 15-90 minutes up to maximum 8 doses.

- Consider intrauterine balloon tamponade for women with bleeding refractory to uterotonics.
- Surgical intervention is recommended including curettage, uterine compression sutures, artery ligation, uterine artery embolization, or hysterectomy if bleeding is refractory to uterotonics and other conservative interventions.

o For PPH due to retained placenta:

- Administer oxytocin IV or IM in combination with controlled cord traction to encourage placental expulsion.
- Attempt manual extraction of placenta followed by single dose of antibiotics (ampicillin or first-generation cephalosporin).
- Consider uterine-conserving surgical extraction (curettage, use of ring forceps) for retained whole placenta.
- Consider hysterectomy sooner rather than later for abnormally adherent (accrete, increta, or percreta).

o For PPH due to damage to the genital tract:

- Repair lacerations to cervix, vagina, or perineum if present.
- Perform I&D for genital tract hematomas and consider packing the vagina.
- Perform exploratory laparotomy for uterine rupture to determine if primary repair is possible or if hysterectomy is necessary.
- For uterine inversion:

- ❖ Attempt manual replacement for inverted uterus with or without uterine relaxants, followed by continuous oxytocin infusion to ensure uterus remains contracted.
- ❖ If nonsurgical correction fails, perform laparotomy.

  o For PPH due to clotting disorders, administer blood products as indicated.
  o Hysterectomy may be indicated for massive hemorrhage unresponsive to other interventions.
  o After resolution of PPH, patient will need iron supplementation for treatment of anemia.

Folic Acid Supplementation in Pregnancy

- Folic acid is given to prevent neural defect (e.g. Spina bifida).
- For low-risk women:

    o Those with planned pregnancy and no personal health risks.
    o 0.4-1 mg daily folic acid for at least 2-3 months before conception and throughout pregnancy and postpartum period.

- For high-risk women:

    o Those with health risks including epilepsy, type 1 DM, BMI > 35, and family history of neural tube defect (NTD).
    o Daily supplementation with multivitamin with 5 mg folic acid for at least 3 months prior to conception until 10-12 weeks post conception.
    o 0.4-1 mg of folic acid from week 12 post conception until postpartum period.

Section 13: Ophthalmology

Allergic Conjunctivitis

- Allergic conjunctivitis is an allergic reaction in the ocular and periocular tissues manifesting as eye redness wit hitching and swelling due to exposure to allergens.
- Seasonal and perennial allergic conjunctivitis have no corneal involvement and result from IgE-mediated hypersensitivity reactions.
- It is usually associated with other manifestations of atopic disease such as allergic rhinitis, asthma, urticaria, and/or atopic dermatitis.
- It usually presents with mild-to-moderate eye redness, tearing, and itching and moderate-to-severe conjunctival swelling (chemosis) in a seasonal or perennial pattern. The initial diagnosis is usually made in late childhood or young adulthood.
- Clinical Features and Diagnosis:

    o The diagnosis is clinical and may be considered in patients with ocular redness (including conjunctival injection), ocular itching, and/or conjunctival swelling, and exposure to a known or suspected allergen.
    o Lab testing is rarely necessary, but an evaluation of conjunctival samples may be considered for patients with severe purulent discharge, refractory disease, or a suspicion of other conditions.
    o Consider a referral to an allergist if the symptoms are not well-controlled for specific allergen testing, such as in vitro tests for specific IgE antibodies, or skin prick and intradermal tests, to support the diagnosis and to guide further therapy.

- Management:

    o Consider a conservative treatment for mild disease, including counseling the patient to avoid rubbing eyes, allergens, and irritants, as well as the benefits of cold compresses and artificial tears.

- Medications may be used for moderate-to-severe disease or for additional symptom relief.

    - Consider dual-action mast cell stabilizer/antihistamine as initial therapy, such as Ketotifen eye drops.
    - Consider single-action medications if the patient is sensitive to the components of dual-action therapy. Antihistamine is contraindicated in patients at risk for angle-closure glaucoma.

        - Antihistamine options include pheniramine maleate, and epinastine eye drops.
        - Mast cell stabilizer options include nedocromil and cromolyn eye drops.

    - Other ocular medications may be considered of the initial therapy is not effective, including topical NSAIDs alone or as an adjunct medication, ocular decongestants as an adjunct treatment, or ocular steroids for unusually severe or resistant cases or if there is a prolonged/repeated exposure to the allergens.

- If prominent allergic rhinitis symptoms are present, consider intranasal steroids, oral antihistamines, and/or oral montelukast.
- Consider a referral to an ophthalmologist if there are significant comorbidities, corticosteroids are needed, or new ocular symptoms develop.

Infective Conjunctivitis

- Infectious conjunctivitis (inflammation of the conjunctiva due to viral or bacterial infection) is usually self-limiting, and rarely results in serious complications.
- Adenovirus is the most common cause, but bacteria (Hemophilus influenza and Streptococcus pneumonia) are also common causes in children.
- Clinical Features and Diagnosis:

    o Suspect infectious conjunctivitis in patient with conjunctival injection (red eye), ocular discharge, and possibly abnormal ocular sensation (itching, burning, or foreign body sensation).

    o Factors that suggest a higher likelihood of bacterial conjunctivitis include gluey or sticky eyes in the morning, mucopurulent discharge, age < 6 years, and absence of itching or burning sensation, though no single factor or pattern is definitive.

    o Refer patient to an ophthalmologist promptly if there is pain, photophobia, visual loss, corneal involvement, or hyperpurulent discharge (gonococcal conjunctivitis).

    o Obtain a conjunctival smear and cultures if there is suspected infectious neonatal conjunctivitis or suspected gonococcal conjunctivitis at any age.

- Management:

    o For presumed viral (or known adenoviral) conjunctivitis:

        - Inform patients that the condition is highly contagious and provide advice to reduce the risk of spread to the other eye or other people.

- Consider symptomatic treatments with artificial tears, topical antihistamines, or cold compresses.

o For acute bacterial conjunctivitis:

- Consider topical antibiotics to improve the rate of early clinical remission, or delayed antibiotics to allow for spontaneous resolution but reduce repeat clinic visits.
- Topical antibiotic options include:

  ❖ Ciprofloxacin ointment 3 times daily for 1 week.
  ❖ Azithromycin twice daily for 2 days, then 1 drop daily for 5 days.
  ❖ Sulfacetamide ointment 4 times daily plus bedtime for 1 week.
  ❖ Trimethoprim/polymyxin B 1-2 drops 4 times daily for 1 week.

o For herpes simplex virus (HSV) conjunctivitis, prescribe antiviral treatment (such as topical ganciclovir 0.15% gel 3-5 times daily or oral famciclovir 250 mg twice daily).

o For gonococcal conjunctivitis, treat with systemic antibiotics (such as ceftriaxone 1 g IM as single dose in adults, or 25-50 mg/kg [maximum 125 mg] IV or IM in infants) and consider daily follow-up until resolution.

o For chlamydia conjunctivitis, treat with systemic antibiotics (such as azithromycin 1 g orally in single dose for patients ≥ 8 years old or who weigh ≥ 45 kg [99 lbs.], or a 14-day course of erythromycin in children who weigh < 45 kg) and reevaluate patients following treatment.

o Refer patients to an ophthalmologist if the conjunctivitis is not responding to therapy within 7 days or there are signs of more complicated disease.

Section 14: Otolaryngology

Acute Otitis Media

- Acute otitis media (AOM) is an infection of the middle ear characterized by the rapid onset of signs and symptoms of inflammation.
- The infection is usually due to a viral or bacterial pathogen, and viral/bacterial co-infection is common.
- The most frequent bacterial pathogens are Streptococcus pneumonia, H. influenza, and M. catarrhalis.
- Clinical features:

    o It frequently presents with ear pain, which may manifest as ear pulling or rubbing in young preverbal children.
    o Other common symptoms include fever, irritability, and difficulty sleeping.
    o Symptoms of an URTI often precede ear symptoms.
    o AOM in children with tympanostomy tubes typically presents with otorrhea without ear pain.

- Diagnosis:

    o Otoscopy findings are usually sufficient to confirm the diagnosis.
    o Diagnose AOM in a child with any of the following:

        - Moderate-to-severe bulging of the tympanic membrane.
        - New onset of otorrhea not due to acute otitis externa.
        - Mild bulging of the tympanic membrane and recent onset of ear pain or intense erythema of the tympanic membrane.

    o AOM should not be diagnosed in the absence of middle ear effusion (based on otoscopy).
    o Consider tympanocentesis for AOM with repeated treatment failure.

- Management:

    o Assess and treat pain; oral analgesics (ibuprofen or acetaminophen).
    o Antibiotics:

       - Are usually indicated for infants < 6 months old and children at increased risk for complication, children with AOM, and moderate to severe otalgia, or febrile > 39 C.
       - Amoxicillin is used for most children (or amoxicillin-clavulanate).
       - Consider cephalosporin if allergic to penicillin.
       - Consider an antibiotic duration of 5 to 10 days, depending on age and AOM severity.

    o Reassess if symptoms worsen or fail to improve within 48-72 hours.
    o Tympanostomy tubes may be considered for children with recurrent AOM, but should not be offered to children with recurrent AOM who don't have middle ear effusion in either ear, unless they are at risk for speech, language, or learning problems, or immunosuppressed.

Section 15: Pediatrics

Acute Epiglottitis

- Acute epiglottitis is a life-threatening condition characterized by upper airway inflammation and obstruction that may occur at any age.
- In children, acute epiglottitis is most commonly due to rapidly progressive bacterial infection, but it may also have a viral or non-infectious (such as trauma) cause.
- The most common causative organisms are beta-hemolytic streptococci (most frequently group A) and Hemophilus influenza type b (Hib).
- Clinical features include:

    o High fever, severe sore throat, and odynophagia accompanied by drooling.
    o Additional manifestations more commonly seen in children include cough, inspiratory stridor, difficulty breathing and dyspnea, muffled phonation/dysphonia, and a toxic appearance.
    o Additional manifestations more commonly seen in adults include change in voice and neck tenderness.
    o If airway obstruction is suspected, avoid using a tongue depressor in physical exam.

- *Differential diagnosis include*: croup, foreign body aspiration, bacterial tracheitis, and trauma.
- Diagnosis:

    o In the presence of respiratory distress, diagnostic procedures should be delayed and priority should be given to securing the airway.
    o In less acute situations, a lateral neck x-ray may confirm suspected acute epiglottitis. The classic radiologic feature is the "thumb" sign, defined as swelling or severe inflammation of the epiglottitis which may lead to irrevocable loss of airway.

- Management:

    o Patients with signs of respiratory distress or upper airway obstruction should be treated as an immediate medical and airway management emergency.
    o Endotracheal/nasotracheal intubation or tracheostomy may be necessary; and prophylactic intubation (not waiting for impending airway obstruction) is recommended in children.
    o Use broad-spectrum second or third generation cephalosporins in combination with penicillinase-resistant penicillin as typical empiric therapy.
    o Consider using IV or aerosol corticosteroid to limit pharyngeal edema and airway obstruction, but there is no high quality evidence that it affects the outcome.
    o Avoid racemic epinephrine as it may result in a rebound effect of rapid and fulminating airway obstruction.

Transient Synovitis (TS)

- Transient synovitis is the most common cause of acute hip pain in children aged 3-10 years.
- The disease causes arthralgia and arthritis secondary to a transient inflammation of the synovium of the hip.
- No definitive cause of TS is known, although the following have been suggested:

    o Patients with TS often have histories of trauma, which may be a predisposing factor.
    o Post-vaccine or drug-mediated reactions and allergic disposition may be a cause.

- Clinical features include:

    o Unilateral hip or joint pain is the most common symptoms reported.
    o Some patient may report medial thigh or knee pain, or present with limp only.
    o Very young children with transient synovitis may have no symptoms other than crying at night.
    o Recent history of URTI, pharyngitis, or otitis media is elicited from half of patients with TS.
    o Physical examination may reveal antalgic limp, and restriction of motion.
    o The most sensitive test for TS is the log roll, in which the patient lies supine and the examiner gently rolls the involved limb from side to side.

- Diagnosis:

  - WBC and ESR may be slightly elevated. High CRP is associated with septic hip arthritis.
  - Ultrasound demonstrates an effusion that causes bulging of the anterior joint capsule.
  - Biopsy reveals only nonspecific inflammation and hypertrophy of the synovial membrane.

- Differential diagnosis includes:

  - Juvenile arthritis.
  - Osteomyelitis.
  - Pediatric septic arthritis.

- Management:

  - Apply heat and massage. Skin traction of the hip in $45°$ of flexion minimizes intracapsular pressure. TS is a self-limited disorder.
  - Treatment with ibuprofen may shorten the duration of symptoms. Advice bed-rest for 7-10 days. Advice the patient not to bear weight on the affected limb, and to avoid full-unrestricted activity until the limb and pain have resolved.

- Complications:

  - Sequelae include coxa magna and mild degenerative changes of the femoral neck.
  - Coxa magna is observed radiographically as an overgrowth of the femoral head and broadening of the femoral neck. Coxa magna lead to dysplasia of the acetabular roof and subluxation.

Croup

- Croup is a common pediatric viral respiratory tract illness, also known as acute laryngotracheitis and acute laryngotracheobronchitis.
- It is generally affects the larynx and trachea, although this illness may also extend to the bronchi.
- Inflammation and edema of the subglottic larynx and trachea, especially near the cricoid cartilage, are the most clinically significant.
- Infective agents are parainfluenza type 1, 2, 3.
- Risk factor includes:

    o Age 3 moths to 5 years, Most common in winter.

- Clinical features include:

    o Inspiratory stridor, worse at night, gradual resolution over 1 week.
    o Seal-like barking cough.
    o Hoarseness.
    o Low grade fever.

- Diagnosis:

    o Mostly clinical diagnosis.
    o X-ray no needed (steeple sign or inverted V shape if an x-ray is performed).

- Management:

    o Treatment is basically supportive and it is treatable at home.

- Cool mist from a humidifier and/or sitting with the child in a bathroom (not in the shower) filled with steam generated by running hot water from the shower, help minimize symptoms.
- Treat fever with antipyretics such as acetaminophen or ibuprofen.

o For severe cases, nebulized racemic epinephrine followed by corticosteroids.

- A single dose of dexamethasone (0.6 mg/kg) is effective in relieving the symptoms, not to exceed 16 mg per day.

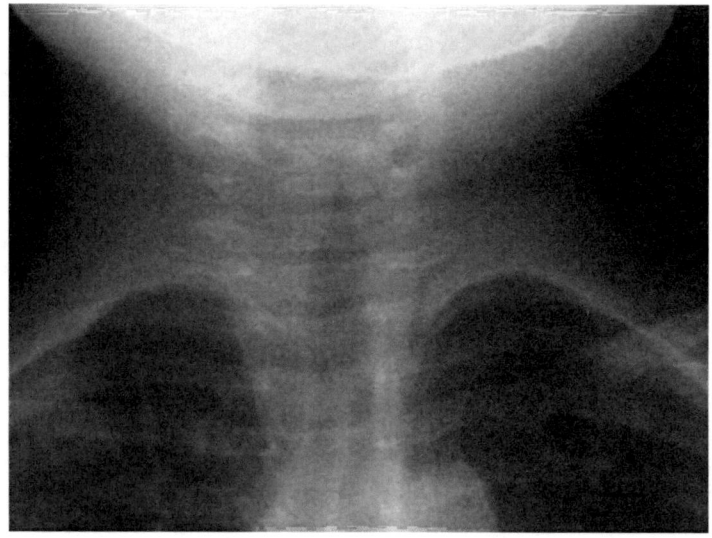

Bronchitis

- Bronchitis is characterized by inflammation of the bronchial tubes (bronchi), the air passages that extend from the trachea into the small airways and alveoli.
- Causes:

    o Hemophilus influenza type B (HiB) no longer number one (due to available vaccine).
    o Streptococcus pyogenes, Streptococcus pneumonia, Staphylococcus aureus, Mycoplasma.

- Risk factors include:

    o Adult or un-immunized child.
    o Usual age range from 2 to 7 years.

- Clinical features:

    o Acute, sudden onset respiratory distress.
    o Extremely sore throat, the patient cannot swallow.
    o High-grade fever.
    o Sniffing position.
    o Drooling.
    o Toxic-appearance.
    o Stridor is a late finding (near-complete obstruction).

- Diagnosis:

    o Clinical first (do nothing to upset child).
    o Controlled visualization (laryngoscopy) of cherry-red, swollen epiglottitis.

- o X-ray is not needed (thumb sign if x-ray is performed).

- **Management:**

  - o Establish patent airway (intubate).
  - o Don't use empiric Antibiotics to cover infective organisms (e.g., Augmentin, Erythromycin).

- **Complications:**

  - o Pneumonia.
  - o Complete airway obstruction and death.

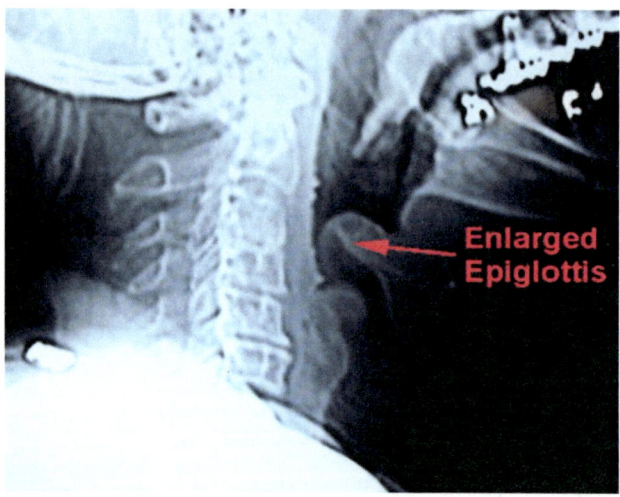

Bronchiolitis

- Bronchiolitis is a viral respiratory infection (usually respiratory syncytial virus "RSV") characterized by an upper respiratory prodrome followed by wheezing and increased respiratory effort in children between 3 months and 2 years old.
- It is the most common LRTI in infants.
- Clinical features include:

  o Wheezing.
  o Fever.
  o Stuffiness, runny nose, mild cough.
  o Tachypnea.
  o Retractions.
  o Increased respiratory effort.

- Diagnosis:

  o Bronchiolitis is diagnosed clinically.
  o Lab tests, radiologic studies, and rapid viral testing not done routinely.
  o Chest X-ray may show hyperinflation with patchy atelectasis.

- Differential diagnosis:

  o Consider pneumonia in children with fever > 39 degrees C.
  o Asthma.
  o Foreign body aspiration.

- Management:
  o Usually supportive treatment:

- Assess hydration and the ability to take fluids orally.
- Use superficial nasal suctioning if necessary.
- Provide supplemental Oxygen if SpO2 is persistently < 90% to maintain SpO2 > 90%.
- Consider nasal continuous positive airway pressure to reduce respiratory distress and hypercapnia.

o Other bronchodilators, corticosteroids, ribavirin, antibiotics, and chest physiotherapy should NOT be used routinely in the management of bronchiolitis.

Kawasaki Disease

- Kawasaki disease was previously referred to as mucocutaneous lymph node syndrome; it is an acute, self-limited, systemic vasculitis of unknown etiology.
- Risk factors include:

  o The majority of affected patients are younger than 5 years.
  o Boys are more frequently affected.

- Diagnostic criteria include:

  o Fever for more than 5 days and at least 4 of the following features:
    - Bilateral, painless, non-exudative conjunctivitis.
    - Lip cracking and fissuring, strawberry tongue, inflammation of the oral mucosa.
    - Cervical lymphadenopathy > 1.5 cm in diameter and usually unilateral.
    - Exanthema.
    - Redness and swelling of the hands and feet with subsequent desquamation.

- Complications include:

  o Myocarditis, pericarditis, valvular heart disease (usually mitral or aortic regurgitation), and coronary arteritis.
  o Those at greatest risk of aneurysm formation are boys, children under the age of 6 months, and those not treated with IVIG.

- Diagnosis:

- o The gold standard for diagnosing coronary artery aneurysm is angiography; however, 2-dimensional echo is highly sensitive and is the current standard screening test in children with Kawasaki disease.

- Management:

  - o The principle goal of treatment is to prevent coronary artery disease and to relieve symptoms.
  - o IVIG 2 g/kg in a single infusion as soon as the diagnosis is made.
  - o Aspirin 80-100 mg/kg/day in 4 divided doses for 14 days or until afebrile for 2-3 days, then switch to aspirin 3-5 mg/kg/day and continue until the absence of coronary artery abnormalities is confirmed 6-8 weeks after the start of illness.
  - o Corticosteroids typically in patients un-responsive to standard therapies.
  - o Methotrexate in IVIG-resistant cases, Infliximab in refractory cases with coronary aneurysm.
  - o During the acute and subacute phases of the illness, patients should be monitored closely by serial ECG, chest radiograph, and echocardiography.

Scarlet Fever

- It is a syndrome characterized by exudative pharyngitis, fever, and bright-red exanthem.
- It is caused by streptococcal pyrogenic exotoxins (SPEs) types A, B, and C.

    o Streptococci are gram-positive cocci.

- Scarlet fever may follow streptococcal wound infections or burins, as well as URTI.
- The person-to-person spread by means of respiratory droplets is the most common mode of transmission. It can rarely spread through contaminated food.
- The incubation period for scarlet fever ranges from 12 hours to 7 days. Patients are contagious during the acute illness and during the subclinical phase.
- Scarlet fever predominantly occurs in children aged 1-10 years. It is rare in children younger than 1 year because of the presence of maternal antiexotoxin antibodies and lack or prior sensitization.
- Clinical features:

    o Fever, associated with sore throat, headache, chills, nausea, myalgia, and malaise.
    o Young children may also present with vomiting, abdominal pain, and seizure.
    o The characteristic rash appears 12-48 hours after the onset of fever, first on the neck and then extending to the trunk and extremities.
    o PE may reveal tender anterior cervical lymphadenopathy, and white strawberry tongue.
    o The mucous membranes are bright red, and scattered petechiae on the soft palate.

- Differential diagnosis include:

    o Rubella (but it has conjunctivitis, purulent rhinitis).
    o Erythema infectiosum, Kawasaki disease, toxic shock syndrome.

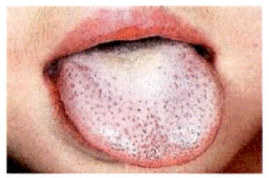

- The diagnosis is mostly based on the clinical presentation.

    o Blood workup can reveal leukocytosis, with a differential of up to 95% polymorphonuclear lymphocytes. During the 2nd week, eosinophilia, as high as 20%, can develop.
    o Throat or nasal culture or rapid streptococcal test is indicated in scarlet fever.

- The goals in treatment of scarlet fever are:

    o To prevent acute rheumatic fever.
    o To reduce the spread of infection.
    o To prevent post-streptococcal glomerulonephritis and suppurative sequelae (e.g. adenitis, mastoiditis, ethmoiditis, and cellulitis).

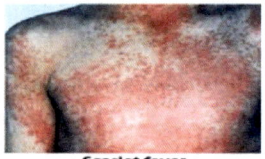

Scarlet fever

- Management:

    o Penicillin (or Amoxicillin) remains the treatment of choice.

        ▪ Dose is 500 mg PO BID, or 250 mg q 6 hours for 10 days.

    o A 1st generation cephalosporin may be an effective alternative (e.g. Cephalexin).
    o If the patient has anaphylactic reactions to penicillin, clindamycin or erythromycin may be considered as an alternative.

- o If odynophagia accompanying streptococcal pharyngitis is especially severe, hospitalization may be warranted for IV hydration and antibiotics.

- Patient education:

  - o Patients should be warned that they will have generalized exfoliation over the next 2 weeks.
  - o They should be warned about the signs of complications of streptococcal infection, such as persistent fever, increased throat or sinus pain, and generalized swelling.

Cystic Fibrosis (CF)

- Cystic fibrosis is transmitted as an autosomal-recessive trait.
- CF is caused by mutations or variants in the CF transmembrane conductance regulator (CFTR) gene.
- The disorder manifests by increased secretions in the upper and lower airways, involves exocrine glands and affects predominantly the GI and respiratory systems.
- Clinical features include:

    o Abdominal distension.
    o Increased frequency of stool.
    o Failure to thrive (despite adequate appetite).
    o Recurrent abdominal pain, Jaundice, GI bleeding.

- Diagnosis:

    o The diagnosis is made by the pilocarpine iontophoresis sweat test:

        - Sweat chloride concentration > 60 mEq/L on 2 occasions confirms diagnosis.
        - Sweat chloride concentration > 30 mEq/L is considered intermediate and requires further evaluation.

- Management:

    o Maintain lung function as near to normal as possible by controlling respiratory infection and clearing airways of mucus.
    o Administer nutritional therapy (i.e., enzyme supplements, multivitamin and mineral supplements) to maintain adequate growth.

- o Offer ivacaftor (Kalydeco) to patients with at least 1 G551D CFTR mutation to improve lung function and quality of life, and to reduce exacerbations.
- o Consider lumacaftor/ivacaftor 200 mg/125 mg (Orkambi) for treatment of CF in patients > 12 years old with F508del mutation.
- o Use dornase alfa (Pulmozyme) to reduce exacerbations in patients with moderate to severe lung disease.

- Complications include:

  - o Meconium ileus present at birth.
  - o Pancreatic insufficiency with possible development of insulin-dependent diabetes.
  - o Retarded growth, Infertility, COPD.
  - o Death usually results from pulmonary complications such as infections with S. aureus, Pseudomonas aeruginosa, and H. influenza.

Hand, Foot, and Mouth Disease

- Hand, foot, and mouth disease (HFMD) is a clinical syndrome characterized by an oral enanthem and a macular, maculopapular, or vesicular rash of the hands and feet (and possibly other locations).
- Coxsackievirus A 16 and enterovirus A 71 are the serotypes most frequently associated with HFMD.
- The viruses that cause HFMD usually are transmitted from person to person by the fecal-oral route. However, they also can be transmitted by contact with oral and respiratory secretions, and vesicle fluid.
- The incubation period for HFMD typically is 2 to 7 days.
- Most cases of HFMD occur in infants and children, particularly those younger than 5 to 7 years.
- *Clinical features include:*

  o Mouth or throat pain (in verbal children), or refusal to eat (in non-verbal children).
  o Fever.
  o The cardinal findings of HFMD are the oral enanthem:

    - The oral lesions of HFMD are anterior to the faucial pillars, most commonly on the tongue and buccal mucosa; less commonly in the gingivolabial groove and on the soft and hard palates.

  o Exanthema:

    - The exanthem associated with HFMD may be macular, maculopapular, or vesicular. All three lesions may occur in a single patient.
    - The exanthem typically involves the hands (dorsum of the fingers, interdigital area, palms), feet (dorsum of the toes,

lateral border of the feet, soles, heels), buttocks, legs (upper thighs), and arms.

- o The skin lesions of HFMD are non-pruritic. They usually are not painful.

- *Complications of HFMD may include:*

  - o Decreased oral intake, which may result in dehydration and may necessitate hospitalization for parenteral fluid therapy.

- The diagnosis of HFMD usually is made clinically.
- *Differential diagnosis* of HFMD includes other conditions associated with oral lesions:

  - o Aphthous ulcers (painful, shallow oral ulcerations with a greyish base, no skin lesions).
  - o Primary herpes simplex gingivostomatitis (oral changes initially consist of erythema and edema of the gingiva with clusters of vesicle.
  - o Contact dermatitis.
  - o Erythema multiforme major (the immune-mediated skin lesions of erythema multiforme have a characteristic target or bull's eye-like appearance.
  - o Eczema herpeticum.

- *Clinical course:*

  - o HFMD generally is a mild clinical syndrome. Complete resolution of symptoms and signs typically occurs within 7 to, at most, 10 days.
- *Management:*

  - o Management is mainly supportive.
  - o Pain and discomfort due to fever can be managed with ibuprofen or acetaminophen (these agents should be avoided in children with dehydration until volume correction has been achieved).

- o In severe cases, oral opioids may be required.
- o Topical oral therapies containing lidocaine are not recommended.

- *Prevention:*

  - o Infants and children with active lesions of HFMD should be excluded from daycare facilities. Strict adherence to hand hygiene protocols is important when changing diapers because enteroviruses are shed in the stool for weeks following infection.
  - o Isolation for hospitalized patients.

- *Indications for hospitalization:*

  - o Inability to maintain adequate hydration.
  - o Development of neurologic or cardiovascular complications such as encephalitis, meningitis, flaccid paralysis, myocarditis.

Tetralogy of Fallot

- Tetralogy of Fallot is a cyanotic congenital heart disease, consisting of 4 heart defects that are present at birth:

    o Pulmonary stenosis.
    o Over-riding aorta.
    o Ventricular septal defect.
    o Right ventricular hypertrophy.

- Diagnosis is suspected based on the presence of heart murmur (harsh systolic murmur), cyanosis, chromosomal abnormality, boot-shaped heart on chest x-ray, right axis deviation and right ventricular hypertrophy on ECG.
- Diagnosis is confirmed by echocardiography.
- Management is done by placing the infant in the knee to chest position in order to prevent hypercyanotic episodes caused by increased pulmonary vascular resistance, preoperative prostaglandin E1 in neonates with severe pulmonary outflow tract obstruction to keep the ductus arteriosus patent and allow adequate pulmonary blood flow, and definitive treatment by surgical closure of the ventricular septal defect.

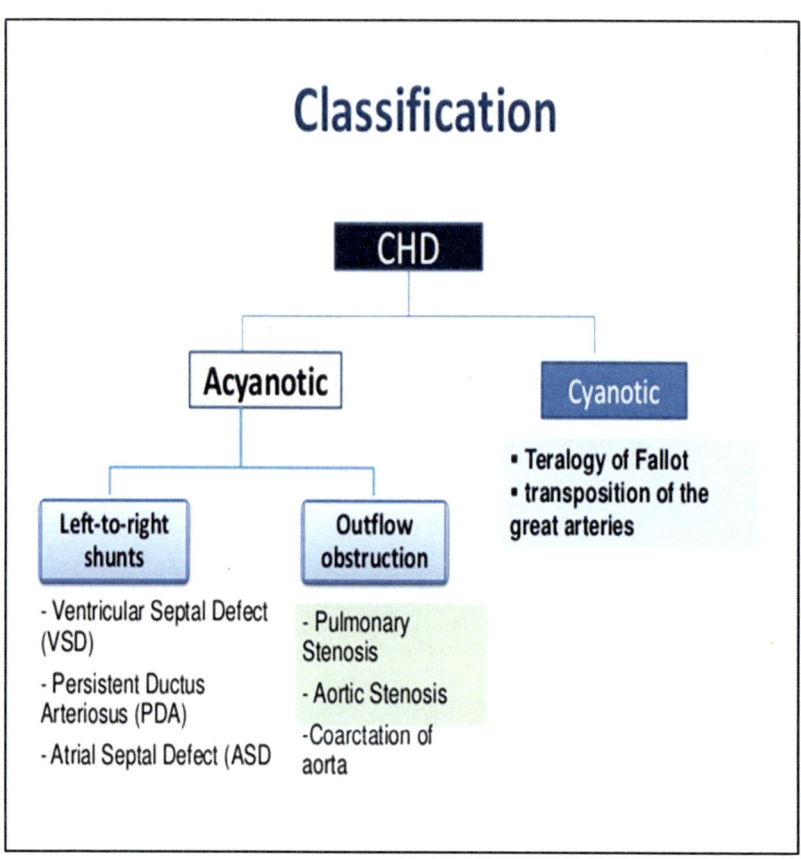

Coarctation of the Aorta

- Coarctation of the aorta is one of the more common congenital heart defects (CHDs).
- Boys are more commonly affected than girls.
- Pathophysiology:

    o The condition occurs when there is discrete narrowing of the thoracic aorta near the ligamentum arteriosus, leading to proximal hypertension and let ventricular overload. Other findings include a VSD, PDA, and bicuspid aortic valve.
    o In infants the condition may be asymptomatic until closure of ductus arteriosus, and then becomes symptomatic with poor perfusion, low cardiac output, or complete cardiovascular collapse.

- Clinical features include:

    o Diminished or absent femoral pulses.
    o Blood pressure higher in the arms than in the legs in infants older than 1 year.
    o 2/6 to 3/6 systolic ejection murmur heard over the apex and upper left sternal border.
    o Left ventricular hypertrophy.

- Diagnosis:

    o Diagnosis is based on physical findings and echocardiography or with CT or MRI angiography.
    o Rib notching on chest radiograph (which is a result of enlargement of the intercostal arteries).

- Management:

    - Initial management in symptomatic newborns involves giving prostaglandin E1 (0.05-0.15 mcg/kg/min is infused IV) to maintain or reopen the ductus arteriosus, as well as resuscitative efforts to correct cardiogenic shock, including inotropic support, ventilator, and fluid resuscitation.
    - In symptomatic children, give diuretics for heart failure. For hypertension, plan prompt surgical relief rather than starting antihypertensive medications.
    - In stable patients, beta blockers and afterload-reducing agents (such as ACE) can be used to postpone definitive treatment until the child is 3 to 5 years of age, when the treatment can be performed electively.
    - Surgical options include transcatheter treatment (balloon angioplasty or stent placement).

Attention Deficit Hyperactivity Disorder (ADHD)

- ADHD is a chronic neurobehavioral disorder consisting of a pattern of inattention or hyperactivity-impulsivity more frequent and severe than typically observed in individuals comparable.
- Risk factors include:

    o Family history of ADHD.
    o Prematurity.
    o Low birth weight.
    o Intrauterine growth restriction.
    o History of brain injury.

- Etiology:

    o The underlying cause may be an abnormality in the central dopaminergic and noradrenergic pathways.

- Clinical features:

    o Children will usually present with a number of behavioral, social, and academic concerns.
    o Physical examination may be normal or show subtle neurologic findings such as imprecise movements.

- Diagnosis:

    o Evaluate all children and adolescents aged 4-18 years presenting with clinical features of ADHD.
    o The DSM-5 diagnostic criteria is one method for making the diagnosis of ADHD:

- Symptoms are present for ≥ 6 months, begin before 12 years, clearly interfere with function, are inappropriate for developmental level with several symptoms being present in > 2 settings, and not better explained by an alternative disorder.
- Children and adolescents < 17 years old have ≥ 6 symptoms from the specific subtype category to diagnose ADHD inattention or hyperactivity/impulsivity subtypes (adolescents aged ≥ 17 years require ≥ 5 symptoms).

Inattention (6 or more)	Hyperactivity/Impulsivity (6 or more)
Fails to attend to details	Blurts out answers
Has difficulty sustaining attention	Difficulty awaiting turn
Does not seem to listen	Interrupts or intrudes
Fails to finish	Talks excessively
Has Difficulty organizing tasks	Fidgets with hands or feel
Avoids sustained effort	Leaves seat in classroom
Loses things	Runs about or climbs
Is distracted by extraneous stimuli	Difficulty laying quietly
Is forgetful	Motor Excess

- Differential diagnosis:

  - Learning or language disorders.
  - Neurodevelopmental disorders.
  - Psychological and behavioral conditions.
  - Sleep disorders.
  - Autism spectrum disorder.

- Management (according to American Academy of Pediatrics):

  - AAP recommendations for children aged 4-5 years:

    - Initial treatment is parent or teacher administered behavioral therapy.

- Consider methylphenidate only if the behavioral interventions don't lead to improvement and if there is moderate to severe functional disturbance.

o AAP recommendations for children aged 6-11 years:

- Treatment with short-acting methylphenidate, extended-release dexmethylphenidate (Focalin), amphetamines (Adderall, Adderall XR), lisdexamfetamine (Vyvanse), or modafinil.
- Parent or teacher-based behavioral therapy.

o AAP recommendations for adolescents aged 12-18 years:

- Treatment with long-acting methylphenidate, extended-release dexmethylphenidate, or lisdexamfetamine.
- Behavioral therapy.

o Non-stimulant medications may be used as a second-line treatment or in addition to other ADHD medication:

- Consider atomoxetine (Strattera) or alpha-2 adrenergic agonists (clonidine or guanfacine) if stimulant medication is ineffective or poorly tolerated.
- Additional options include carbamazepine or antidepressants.

o Consider follow-up every 1-3 weeks for initial dose titration, then every 3-6 months.
o Other measures to consider include neurofeedback and zinc supplementation.
o A screening ECG before starting stimulant medications has been suggested by the AHA, but not the AAP.

Encopresis

- Encopresis is the involuntary discharge of feces, usually older than 4 years (i.e., fecal incontinence).
- Classifications:

  o Retentive encopresis:

    ▪ It is more common, seen both with chronic constipation and overflow incontinence.

  o Non-retentive encopresis:

    ▪ Encopresis without constipation.

- Clinical features:

  o Constipation, painful defecation, inability to differentiate passing gas and passing feces, and soiling episodes usually occurring during daytime.
  o Physical examination may reveal palpable stool throughout the distribution of the colon, stool smeared around the anus, lax anal sphincter.

- Diagnosis:

  o The radiograph demonstrates a dilated, stool-filled colon consistent with retentive encopresis.

- Differential diagnosis:

  o Spina bifida, Meningomyelocele, Spinal-cord injury with dysfunctional of the anal sphincter., Imperforate anus with fistula, Constipation, and rarely Hirschsprung's disease.

- Management:

  o Clearing the fecal mass.
  o Maintaining soft stools for a short period of time with mineral oil or stool softeners (3-6 months).
  o Behavioral modification.

Enuresis

- Enuresis is intermittent involuntary urinary incontinence at least twice weekly while sleeping (at night or during naps) in children > 5 years old.
- Classification:

  o Primary enuresis:

    - Is never having had a dry period > 6 months.
    - Etiology includes genetic predisposition, excessive evening/nighttime fluid intake, constipation, and disordered sleep.

  o Secondary enuresis:

    - Is nighttime wetting in a child previously dry > 6 months.
    - Etiology includes psychological stress or medical disorders such as constipation, cystitis, DM, obstructive sleep apnea, overactive bladder, neurogenic bladder, urethral obstruction, seizure disorder, or diabetes insipidus.

- Clinical features include:

  o Most enuresis is monosymptomatic, but it can also be polysymptomatic in a constellation of voiding symptoms of urgency, frequency, and incontinence.
  o Parent presents with child for concerns about persistent or new nighttime bedwetting.
  o Important historical information includes volume, timing, and pattern of enuresis as well as toilet training history, fluid intake history, bowel/stool history, sleep history, and any associated urinary symptoms.

- Diagnosis:

    o Workup for enuresis is directed by the history and physical.
    o Consider urine dipstick, urine microscopy or culture.

- Management:

    o Identify and treat underlying cause.
    o Offer reassurance that most enuresis resolves over time (15% per year among children > 6 years old).
    o Behavioral treatments include (Fluid restriction 1.5 hours prior to bedtime, enuresis alarm).
    o Medical management includes Desmopressin 0.2-0.4 mg PO 1 hour prior to bedtime (stop desmopressin after 1 week every 3 months to assess for resolution of enuresis).
    o Consider referral to urologist when patient has severe daytime symptoms, a history of recurrent UTI, suspected neurological problems, or lack of response to primary treatment.

Failure to Thrive (FTT)

- Failure to thrive (FTT) is defined as inadequate growth or inability to maintain growth.
- Most quantitative definitions are growth chart-based, but growth curves alone cannot be used to diagnose FTT.
- Examples of quantitative definitions include measurement on multiple occasions showing:

  - BMI for age < 5th percentile.
  - Weight < 5th percentile for sex and corrected age.
  - Weight-for-length < 5th percentile.
  - Sustained fall in weight for age or weight for length/height by 2 major percentiles (defined as 95th, 90th, 75th, 50th, 25th, 10th, and 5th).

- Risk factors include low birth weight, prematurity, congenital anomalies, developmental delay, eosinophilic esophagitis, GERD, poverty, family stressors, and postpartum depression.
- FTT is caused by inadequate nutrition, with no underlying medical cause identified in > 80% of patients.
- Common causes include:

  - Inadequate nutritional intake, inadequate nutrition absorption (CF, IBS, anemia, and biliary atresia), increased metabolic demand (hyperthyroidism, TORCH syndrome, and chronic lung disease).

- Clinical Features and Diagnosis:

  - Evaluation consists of detailed nutritional history, family growth history. Assessment of GI symptoms including feeding and stool patterns, and an evaluation of the growth chart.

- History and physical exam should be directed at identifying possible underlying causes.
- Evaluation should include rechecking results of newborn screen.
- Tests to consider if history and physical are nonspecific and growth has not improved with dietary interventions include CBC, chemistry panel, lead level, antibody testing for celiac disease, urinalysis, stool, studies, sweat test to rule out cystic fibrosis (CF), and tuberculin skin test.
- Other tests should primarily be ordered to identify suspected cause suggested by history or physical.

- Management:

  - Give appropriate treatment for any underlying disorder identified.
  - Using calculated energy and protein needs, give sufficient nutritional repletion (including calorie-dense foods) to produce catch-up growth and a return to normal growth curve.
  - Consider supplemental enteral feedings is not achieving catch-up growth or weight gain is slow.
  - Avoid refeeding syndrome (severe electrolyte and fluid shifts that occur when feedings are increased too rapidly in a malnourished patient).
  - Inpatient admission may be indicated for psychosocial issues, serious malnutrition, or failure to improve with outpatient management.

Barlow Maneuver

- It is a physical examination performed on infants to screen for developmental dysplasia of the hip.
- The maneuver is performed by adducting the hip (bringing the thigh toward the midline) while applying light pressure on the knee, directing the force posteriorly.
- If the hip is dislocatable—that is, if the hip can be popped out of socket with this maneuver-the test is considered positive.
- The Ortolani maneuver is then used, to confirm the positive finding.

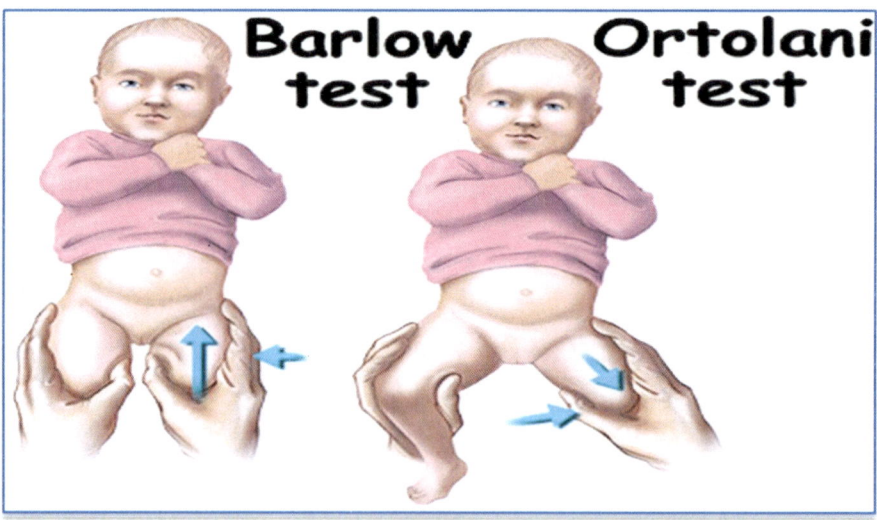

Ortolani Maneuver

- Ortolani test is part of the physical examination for developmental dysplasia of the hip, along with the Barlow maneuver.
- It relocates the dislocation of the hip joint that has just been elicited by the Barlow.
- It is performed by an examiner first flexing the hips and knees of a supine infant to 90 degrees, then with the examiner's index fingers placing anterior pressure on the greater trochanters, gently and smoothly abducting the infant's legs using the examiner's thumbs. A positive sign is a distinctive "clunk" which can be heard and felt as the femoral head relocates anteriorly into the acetabulum. Specifically, this test for posterior dislocation of the hip.

Rickets

- Rickets is a bone disorder that affects growing children; it is characterized by deficient mineralization (calcification) of the growth plate, which can lead to impaired growth and skeletal deformity.
- Abnormal growth plate mineralization is due to deficiencies of calcium and/or vitamin D (resulting in calcipenic rickets), or phosphate (resulting in phosphopenic rickets).
- These deficiencies may be due to:

  - Inadequate intake (nutritional rickets) or malabsorption of calcium, vitamin D, or phosphate, or decreased skin synthesis of vitamin D (because of inadequate sun exposure).
  - Hereditary defects in vitamin D metabolism (vitamin D-dependent rickets type IA and IB) or in end-organ response to vitamin D (vitamin D-dependent rickets type IIA and IIB).
  - Hereditary defects and nonhereditary conditions associated with increased renal loss of phosphate.

- Risk factors for rickets include exclusive breastfeeding or a vegetarian diet without vitamin D supplementation, dark skin or limited sunlight exposure, prematurity, and conditions or medications that impair the absorption or metabolism of calcium, phosphorus, or vitamin D.
- Rickets often presents as bone deformities, poor growth, tetany, seizures, and/or myopathy.
- Evaluations:

  - Suspect rickets in a growing child with any of the following:

    - Enlarged wrists, knees, or ankles, or bowing of weight-bearing extremities.

- A rachitis rosary (enlarged costochondral joints, palpable or visible as bead-like thickenings lateral to the nipple line) or Harrison's groove (flaring of the ribs at the level of the diaphragm).
- Hypocalcemic seizures (suspect nutritional or vitamin D-dependent rickets).
- Pain in the lower limbs or back, muscle weakness in an adolescent, or craniotabes in an infant or young child).

  o Confirm the diagnosis by:

  - An anteroposterior X-ray of a rapidly growing skeletal area (for example, the knee or wrist) showing widened growth plates with metaphyseal cupping and irregularity.
  - Blood tests showing decreased phosphate, increased ALP, normal or decreased calcium, and normal BUN and creatinine levels.

- Management:

  o Treat nutritional rickets with supplementation to correct specific deficiency, such as:

  - Vitamin D recommendations vary with initial dose of vitamin D2 or D3 from 500,000 units (1,250-15,000 mcg) per week, then maintenance dosing 400-1,000 units/day (10-25 mcg/day).
  - Calcium 40-80 mg/kg/day (1-2 mmol/kg/day) orally in 4-6 divided doses.
  - Phosphate 15 mg/kg/day (0.48 mmol/kg/day) orally in 3-4 divided doses.

  o Treat vitamin D-dependent rickets with calcitriol or alphacalcidol (1 alpha-hydroxyvitamin D) orally. For type II vitamin D-dependent rickets, add calcium orally or IV and consider consulting a pediatric nephrologist.

- Treat phosphopenic rickets with both:

    - Phosphorus 20-40 mg/kg/day orally in 3-5 divided doses.
    - Calcitriol 20-30 ng/kg/day orally in 2-3 divided doses, except in hypophosphatemic rickets with hypercalciuria (because vitamin D may increase the risk of nephrocalcinosis and nephrolithiasis).

- Excise the tumor or nevus in rare lesions (tumor-induced rickets or linear nevus sebaceous syndrome) which secrete fibroblast growth factor 23 (FGF-23).

Section 16: Respiratory

Differential Diagnosis of Dyspnea

- Dyspnea, also known as shortness of breath, is difficulty or labored breathing.
- Differential diagnosis of dyspnea include:

  o *Cardiovascular:*
    - Acute MI.
    - CHF/LV failure.
    - Aortic/mitral stenosis.
    - Aortic/mitral regurgitation.
    - Arrhythmia.
    - Cardiac tamponade.
    - Constrictive pericarditis.
    - Left-sided obstructive lesions (e.g., left atrial myxoma).
    - Elevated pulmonary venous pressure.

  o *Respiratory:*
    - Airway disease:
      - Asthma.
      - COPD exacerbation.
      - Upper airway obstruction (anaphylaxis, foreign body, mucus plugging).
    - Parenchymal lung disease:
      - Acute respiratory distress syndrome (ARDS).
      - Pneumonia, Interstitial lung disease.

- Pulmonary vascular disease:
  - PE, Pulmonary HTN, Pulmonary vasculitis.
- Pleural disease:
  - Pneumothorax.
  - Pleural effusion.

o *Neuromuscular and chest wall disorders:*

- C-spine injury.
- Polymyositis, myasthenia gravis, Guillain-Barre syndrome.
- Kyphoscoliosis.

o *Hematological/metabolic:*

- Anemia, acidosis, hypercapnia.

o *Anxiety/psychosomatic:*

Bronchial Asthma

- Asthma is a heterogeneous disease, usually characterized by chronic airway inflammation. It is defined by the history of respiratory symptoms such as wheeze, shortness of breath, chest tightness and cough that vary time and in intensity, together with variable expiratory airflow limitation.

Management:
- Classification of asthma: Mild intermittent (Step1).
- Mild persistent (Step2).
- Moderate persistent (Step3).
- Severe persistent (Step4).

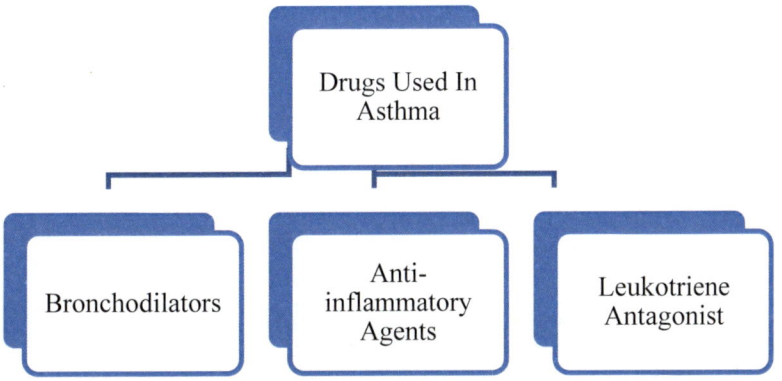

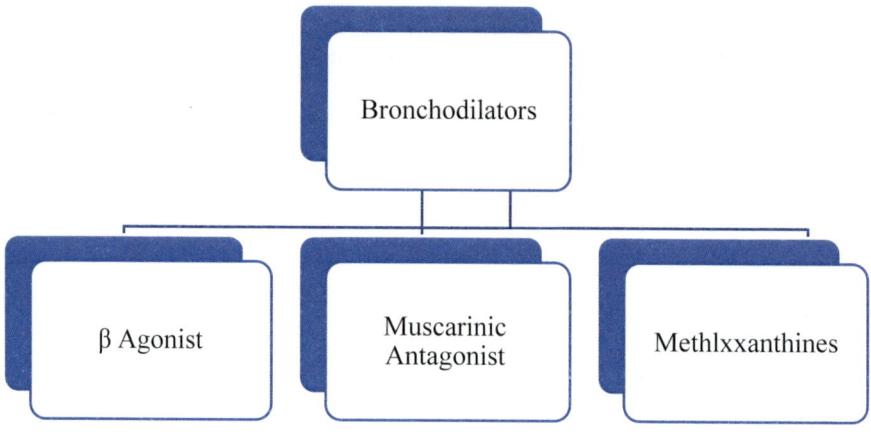

- Beta agonist:

    - Almost given by inhalation, and sometimes by nebulizer.
    - Albuterol, terbutaline and metaproterenol (Short acting – Acute asthma).
    - Stimulate adenyl cyclase (AC), and increase cAMP.
    - Salmeterol and formoterol (Long acting 12 hrs or more – used for prophylaxis and COPD).
    - Side effect: (Tremors – Tachycardia – Arrhythmias – Tolerance).

- Muscarinic Antagonist:

    - Does NOT cause tremor or arrhythmia.
    - Blocks muscarinic receptors.
    - E.g., Ipratropium and Tiotropium.

- Methylxanthines:

    - Inhibit phosphodiesterase (PDE).
    - Found in plants and caffeine.
    - Side effect: (GI distress – Tremor – Insomnia).

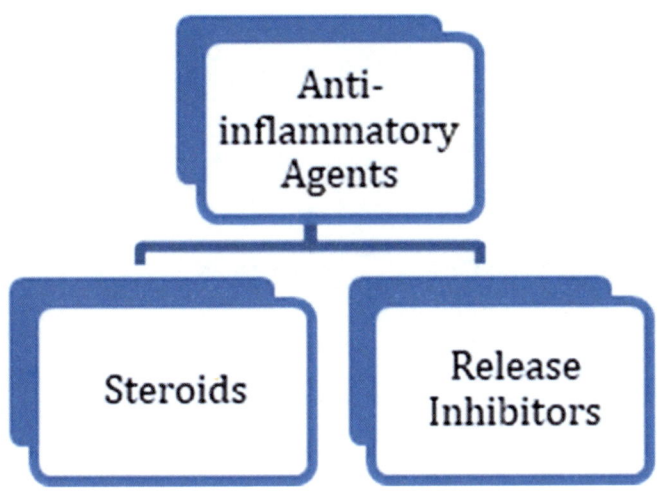

- Corticosteroids:

    - Reduces the synthesis of arachidonic acid.
    - Inhibit cytokine production.
    - E.g., Fluticasone.
    - Inhaled corticosteroid is a first line therapy for moderate to severe asthma.

- Cromolyn & Nedocromil:

    - Decrease the release of mediators (leukotrienes – histamine).
    - Commonly used in children.
    - Drug allergy is rare.

Inhalation	Systemic
Long term prevention	Short term in acute asthma
Reduce need for oral	Long term prevention

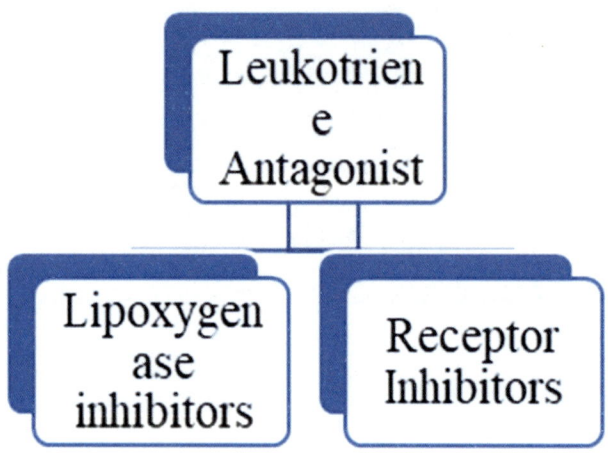

- Leukotriene antagonists:

    - Not recommended for acute asthma.
    - Zileuton: is a selectively inhibits 5-lipoxygenase.
    - Zileuton convert arachidonic acid to LT.
    - NOT as effective as corticosteroid in severe asthma.
    - Zafirlukast and Montelukast are LTD4 receptor antagonist.

Chronic Obstructive Pulmonary Disease (COPD)

- COPD is characterized by significant airflow limitation associated with a chronic inflammatory response in the airways and lungs resulting in the destruction of lung tissue.
- Terms "emphysema" and "chronic bronchitis" not included in Global Initiative for Chronic Obstructive Lung Disease (GOLD) definition of COPD:

    o Chronic bronchitis: cough and excess sputum production for > 3 months per year in each of 2 consecutive years.
    o Emphysema: pathological term describing destruction of gas exchanging surfaces of lung (alveoli).

- It commonly affects adults > 40 years old who smoke.
- Risk factors include:

    o Smoking is the most common risk factors for COPD worldwide.
    o Occupational exposures (e.g., organic and inorganic dusts, chemical agents, and fumes).
    o Alpha-1 antitrypsin deficiency.
    o Indoor air pollution.

- GOLD severity classification of airflow limitation in COPD:

    o Diagnosis of COPD applied to patients with airflow limitation, defined as forced expiratory volume in 1 second (FEV_1)/forced vital capacity (FVC) ratio < 0.7.

Severity	FEV$_1$
GOLD 1 (Mild)	> 80% predicted
GOLD 2 (Moderate)	50%-80% predicted
GOLD 3 (Severe)	30%-50% predicted
GOLD 4 (Very severe)	< 30% predicted

- Clinical features include:

    o Chronic and progressive symptoms of dyspnea, cough, and sputum production.
    o Physical exam may show the use of accessory muscles, reduced chest expansion, wheezing, hyperresonance to percussion, and reduced breath sounds.
    o A physical examination may also help detect the signs of acute exacerbation of COPD, such as central cyanosis, hemodynamic instability, and reduced alertness.

- Diagnosis:

    o Spirometry documenting forced expiratory volume in 1 second (FEV$_1$)/forced vital capacity (FVC) ratio < 0.7 consistent with COPD diagnosis.
    o Additional testing for a patient workup includes measuring oxygen saturation (sometimes followed by an arterial blood gas), a CBC, and a chest X-ray.

- Management:

    o Encourage smoking cessation for patients who smoke.
    o Administer an influenza vaccination annually.
    o Pulmonary rehabilitation (including exercise training, nutrition counseling) is recommended for patients with symptoms and/or high risk of exacerbation.

- In patients with severe, chronic resting hypoxemia (PaO2 < 55 mmHg or oxygen saturation < 88%) offer continuous oxygen therapy.
- Management by disease severity:

Classification	Management
GOLD A	1st line drug therapy is short or long acting bronchodilator
GOLD B	1st line drug therapy is long acting bronchodilator, and add second bronchodilator if symptoms not controlled with monotherapy
GOLD C	1st line drug therapy is long acting bronchodilator, long-acting muscarinic receptor antagonist (LAMA) recommended over LABA, if persistent exacerbations, add LABA or inhaled corticosteroid
GOLD D	1st line drug therapy is LABA/LAMA combination in most patients, but LABA/ICS may be preferred in patients with history of asthma-COPD overlap syndrome

- Inhaled LABA include:
    - Salmeterol 1 inhalation (50 mcg) via dry powder inhaler (DPI) twice daily.
- Inhaled LAMA include:
    - Ipratropium 2 inhalations (17 mcg each) via MDI 4 times daily.
- LABA/LAMA combination inhalers include:
-
    - Vilanterol/Umeclidinium 1 inhalation (25 mcg/62.5 mcg) via DPI once daily.

- ○ ICS at doses equivalent to beclomethasone > 1000 mcg/day for > 6 months.

- Complications of COPD include:

  - ○ Acute exacerbation, respiratory failure, and pulmonary hypertension.

Section 17: Urology

Benign Prostatic Hyperplasia (BPH)

- BPH is a benign enlargement of the prostate gland due to stromal and epithelial cell hyperplasia, and is the most common benign neoplasm in older men.
- BPH leads to lower urinary tract symptoms (LUTS) including obstructive voiding symptoms (weak urinary stream, straining, hesitancy, dribbling) and urine storage (irritative) symptoms (urgency, frequency, nocturia, urge incontinence).
- Diagnosis:

    o Review medications which may be contributing to symptoms such as antihistamines, muscle relaxants, opioids, tricyclic antidepressants, antispasmodics, and sympathomimetic drugs.
    o Perform a digital rectal exam to evaluate rectal tone and prostate size, consistency, shape, and irregularities.
    o Obtain a urine dipstick analysis to identify clues to causes of symptoms other than BPH.
    o It is recommended that the patient complete frequency volume charts if nocturia is a predominant symptom.
    o Refer to urologist for detailed evaluation if there are signs of disease beyond BPH such as a suspicious digital rectal exam, hematuria, abnormal PSA level, pain, recurrent or persistent infection, palpable bladder, or urinary retention.

- Management:

    o Offer watchful waiting for men with mild LUTS due to BPH such as AUA-SI score < 8 and moderate-to-severe LUTS who are not bothered by their symptoms.

- o Consider limiting nocturnal fluid intake, avoiding excess alcohol, and increasing physical activity as lifestyle changes that may reduce LUTS.
- o For patients with moderate-to-severe symptoms of BPH warranting treatment:

    - Offer an alpha-1 blocker:

        - ❖ Use caution if the patient is taking a phosphodiesterase-5 inhibitor, undergoing cataract surgery, or at risk for orthostatic hypotension.

    - Consider a 5-alpha reductase inhibitor if the estimated prostate size is > 30 g or the PSA level is > 1.4 ng/mL.
    - Consider an anticholinergic drug in men with predominantly irritative LUTS without elevated postvoid residual, especially if there is concomitant overactive bladder.
    - For men with nocturnal polyuria, consider furosemide in the late afternoon or desmopressin.

- o Offer surgery for LUTS refractory to other therapies or BPH leading to complications such as renal insufficiency or recurrent UTIs.

    - Surgical options include transurethral resection of the prostate (TURP), transurethral vaporization of the prostate, transurethral incision of the prostate (TUIP) if the estimated prostate size is < 30 g, transurethral laser therapies, and prostatectomy if the estimated prostate size is > 80 g.
    - Most transurethral surgical treatments appear to have similar efficacy for reducing LUTS due to BPH.

- o A prostatic urethral lift (UroLift) has been shown to improve LUTS in men with BPH.
- Complications of BPH include urinary retention, UTI, CKD, neurogenic bladder, and bladder stones.

Disease Severity	AUA Symptom Score	Typical Symptoms and Signs
Mild	≤7	Asymptomatic Peak urinary flow rate <10 mL/s PVR urine volume >25–50 mL
Moderate	8–19	All of the above signs plus obstructive voiding symptoms and irritative voiding symptoms (signs of detrusor instability)
Severe	≥20	All of the above plus one or more complications of BPH

AUA, American Urological Association; BPH, benign prostatic hyperplasia; BUN, blood urea nitrogen; PVR, postvoid residual.

Section 18: Miscellaneous

Dehydration and Fluid Management

- Dehydration is a general term used to describe any type of fluid loss.
- Common causes include fluid loss from the GI tract, skin, kidneys, or third-space sequestration.
- Types of dehydration include:

    o Isotonic (Isonatremic): in which Na level is 135-145 mmol/L.
    o Hypotonic (hyponatremic): in which Na level is < 135 mmol/L.
    o Hypertonic (hypernatremic): in which Na level is > 145 mmol/L.

- Causes of dehydration include:

    o Isotonic dehydration:

        - Hemorrhage, Excessive GI losses, Trauma (including surgical trauma), and Capillary leak syndrome.

    o Hypertonic dehydration:

        - Severe GI losses (including vomiting or diarrhea), limited oral fluid intake, Diuretics, Dermal losses (including burns or sweating), renal disease, and diabetes.

    o Hypotonic dehydration:

        - Renal losses (such as Diuretics, adrenal insufficiency, and salt-wasting nephropathy), and extrarenal sodium loss (such as Vomiting, Dermal losses, and Fluid sequestration).

- Assessment of Dehydration involves:

Deficits ➡	Infants 5% (50 mL/kg) Older Child 3% (30 mL/kg)	10% (100 mL/kg) 6% (60 mL/kg)	15% (150 mL/kg) 9% (90 mL/kg)
Dehydration	**Mild**	**Moderate**	**Severe**
Skin turgor	Normal	Tenting	None
Skin (touch)	Normal	Dry	Clammy
Buccal mucosa/lips	Moist	Dry	Parched/cracked
Eyes	Normal	Deep set	Sunken
Tears	Present	Reduced	None
Fontanelle	Flat	Soft	Sunken
CNS	Consolable	Irritable	Lethargic/obtunded
Pulse rate	Normal	Slightly increased	Increased
Pulse quality	Normal	Week	Feeble/impalpable
Capillary refill	Normal	~ 2 seconds	> 3 seconds
Urine output	Normal	Decreased	Anuric

- Conditions that may lead to dehydration include:

    o Gastroenteritis.
    o Stomatitis (pain may severely limit oral intake).
    o DKA.
    o Pharyngitis (may decrease oral intake).
    o Burns.

- Deficits replacement as:

    o Half volume over 8 hours, and half volume over 16 hours.
    o *EXCEPTION:* hypernatremic dehydration, replace deficit over 48 hours.

- Supplying maintenance fluid requirements in children as follows:

  o 100 mL/kg/day for the first 10 kg of weight (or 4 mL/kg/hour).
  o 50 mL/kg/day for the second 10 kg of weight (or 2 mL/kg/hour).
  o 20 mL/kg/day for each additional kg (or 1 mL/kg/hour).

- General management include:

  o Mild dehydration:
    - Oral rehydration.
    - If mild diarrhea should feed regular diet (may delay 6-12 hours).
    - If vomiting give about 120 ml of ORS (if below 1 year old), or 240 ml (if > 1 year old).
    - Breastfeeding should NOT stop.

  o Moderate dehydration:
    - Oral rehydration.
    - IV (if uncontrolled vomiting, unable to drink because of extreme fatigue, stupor, or coma, or those with gastric or intestinal distension).

  o Severe dehydration:
    - IV rehydration with lactated Ringers or normal saline solution.
    - Consider resuscitation with 20 ml/kg if patient in shock.

Ankle Brachial Index (ABI)

- It is a ratio of systolic blood pressure in ankle to that in brachial artery.
- Interpretation of ABI:
    - More than 1.3 = poorly compressible vessels.
    - 0.9-1.3 = normal.
    - 0.4-0.89 = moderate to mild obstruction.
    - Less than 0.4 = severe obstruction.

Hyperkalemia

- Hyperkalemia is a serum potassium level > 5.5 mmol/L (reference ranges may vary between labs).
- *Classifications:*

  o Mild hyperkalemia:
    - Potassium level 5.5-5.9 mmol/L.

  o Moderate hyperkalemia:
    - Potassium level 6-6.5 mmol/L.

  o Severe hyperkalemia: any of the following:
    - Potassium level > 6.5 mmol/L.
    - ECG changes and potassium level > 5.5 mmol/L.
    - Symptoms of hyperkalemia (including palpitations) and potassium level > 5.5 mmol/L.

- *Causes:*

  o Pathogenesis includes an increased potassium intake above the ability for excretion by the kidneys (or GIT) or shifting from intracellular to extracellular space.

  o Etiology of hyperkalemia most often multifactorial and usually associated with renal failure, tubular dysfunction, or shifting of potassium from intracellular to extracellular space.

  o Impaired renal excretion:

- Acute renal failure, chronic kidney disease, diabetic nephropathy, SLE.

  o Renal tubular acidosis (RTA) type IV hypoaldosteronism:

  - Causes include mineralocorticoid deficiency (e.g. Addison's disease).

  o Potassium redistribution or release into extracellular space:

  - Hyperosmolar states such as hyperglycemia, volume depletion, acidosis.

  o Common sources of exogenous potassium load:

  - Potassium supplements, TPN, RBC transfusion, penicillin G potassium.

- *Clinical features include:*

  o Often asymptomatic, Muscular weakness, flaccid paralysis, Cardiac arrhythmia.
  o Decreased bowel motility (ileus).

- *Differential diagnoses* include pseudohyperkalemia due to lab artifact.

  o Pseudohyperkalemia is due to excessive leakage of potassium from cells during blood is drawn.

- *Diagnosis:*

  o Repeat potassium levels for verification if the patient is asymptomatic and has no obvious risk factors.
  o Consider checking both serum and plasma potassium levels to help distinguish true hyperkalemia from pseudohyperkalemia.

- Check serum electrolytes, calcium, magnesium, BUN, creatinine, and glucose.
- Perform ECG:

    - The earliest ECG changes are peaked, narrow T waves and shortened QT intervals.
    - At plasma potassium concentration > 7 mmol/L, widening QRS complexes, decreased amplitude of P waves, PR prolongation, and 2nd or 3rd degree AV block may be seen.
    - ECG changes can progress to sine wave pattern with widening QRS complex merging with T wave, and eventually lead to ventricular fibrillation or asystole.

- Perform cardiac monitoring if severe hyperkalemia is present.

- *Management:*

    - Urgent treatment is recommended if the patient has potassium levels > 6.5 mmol/L, hyperkalemia associated with ECG changes, symptomatic hyperkalemia, or hyperkalemia in the setting of impaired renal function or significant acidosis.
    - If urgent treatment is indicative, give Calcium gluconate 10-20 mL of 10% solution IV (0.5 mL/kg in children) over 2-3 minutes to stabilize the myocardial conduction system.

        - Repeat the dose as needed. Use with caution in patients taking digoxin due to toxicity.
        - The stabilizing effect of calcium will last 30 to 60 minutes, allowing time for other corrective measures to be taken.

    - Give insulin to shift potassium from the extracellular to the intracellular space:

        - Unless the patient is hyperglycemic, IV glucose is also given to prevent hypoglycemia.

- The usual dose is 10 units of insulin and 25 g of IV glucose (one ampulla of D50).

o Nebulized albuterol can also be used to drive potassium into cells.

- The common dose is 10-20 mg in adults, and 2.5 mg in children.

o Bicarbonate therapy will cause the potassium to shift intracellularly. Given the risks associated with bicarbonate therapy, this therapy is usually reserved for patients who are significantly acidotic and are able to be effectively ventilated.
o Diuretics, such as furosemide 20-40 mg IV, if the patient has adequate renal function (onset of action is 15-60 minutes with action lasting 4 hours).
o Sodium polystyrene sulfonate (Kayexalate) 15 g 1-4 times/day orally in adults will reduce potassium stores in the body (onset of action is 1-2 hours and lasting for 4-6 hours).
o Hemodialysis is utilized in refractory cases, or in chronic kidney disease patients who already have dialysis access.

Hyponatremia

- Hyponatremia is characterized as serum sodium < 135 mmol/L.
- Classifications:

    o Hypotonic hyponatremia, TRUE HYPONATREMIA (serum osmolality < 280 mOsm/kg):

    - *Hypovolemic hyponatremia:* can be caused by GI losses (such as diarrhea or vomiting), renal volume losses (due to diuretics, cerebral salt wasting, and adrenal insufficiency), and dermal losses (such as burns or sweating).
    - *Euvolemic hyponatremia:* is often caused by syndrome of inappropriate antidiuresis (SIAD), but other causes include low solute intake, hypothyroidism, water intoxication, exercise-associated hyponatremia, and glucocorticoid deficiency.
    - *Hypervolemic hyponatremia:* can be caused by heart failure, cirrhosis, and kidney disease.

    o Isotonic hyponatremia (serum osmolality 280-295 mOsm/kg):

    - Can be due to pseudohyponatremia.

    o Hypertonic hyponatremia (serum osmolality > 295 mOsm/kg:

    - Can be due to hypertonic fluid infusion or hyperglycemia.

- Clinical features include:

    o Hypovolemic hyponatremia:

- Patients typically present with clinical symptoms or signs of volume depletion, such as vomiting and diarrhea, orthostatic decreases in blood pressure and increases in pulse rate, dry mucus membranes, and decreased skin turgor.

  o Euvolemic hyponatremia:

  - Patients typically present without clinical signs of volume depletion or expansion.

  o Hypervolemic hyponatremia:

  - Patients typically present with signs of volume overload, such as dependent edema, ascites, or rales (pulmonary edema).

  o Mild hyponatremia:

  - Usually asymptomatic, nausea or malaise may be found.

  o Symptoms with severe or rapid onset hyponatremia may include:

  - Seizures.
  - Coma.
  - Respiratory arrest.

- Diagnosis:

  o Repeat serum sodium levels to confirm the initial reading.
  o Assess volume status in combination with other test results.

- Management:

  o Initial treatment:

- Establish reliable IV access and give supplemental oxygen to patients with lethargy or obtundation.
- Avoid giving hypotonic IV fluid because they may exacerbate cerebral edema.

o Goal of treatment is to:

- Correct serum sodium levels to avoid complications of sever hyponatremia including cerebral edema, seizures, coma, brainstem herniation, respiratory arrest and death.
- Avoid rapid correction of hyponatremia which may result in osmotic demyelination syndrome (central pontine myelinolysis) with symptoms including dysarthria, dysphagia, spastic paraparesis, and lethargy.

o Rate of correction:

- For patients with symptoms of severe hyponatremia, regardless of chronicity, rapid increase in serum sodium by 4-6 mmol/L is recommended. Additional increases may be necessary if symptoms persist after the initial rise in sodium. Don't increase sodium more than 8 mmol/L during the first 24 hours because of the risk of demyelination.
- For asymptomatic or mildly symptomatic patients, a safe rate of sodium correction depends on the duration of hyponatremia:

    ❖ Correct acute hyponatremia (< 24 to 48 hours) without restricting rate of rise. If there is any uncertainty regarding whether hyponatremia is acute or chronic, manage as chronic.
    ❖ For patients with chronic hyponatremia (> 48 hours), increase serum sodium with a goal of < 8 mmol/L/day in usual risk of osmotic demyelination syndrome. High risk osmotic demyelination syndrome (such as

malnutrition, alcoholism, or revere hyponatremia), increase serum sodium with a goal of < 6 mmol/L/day.
- ❖ Monitor serum sodium every 4-6 hours during correction.

- o Management options include:
    - For patients with symptomatic severe hyponatremia, regardless of duration and etiology, give 100 mL of 3% saline solution as an IV infusion.
    - For patients with hypovolemic hyponatremia, correct volume depletion with IV isotonic (0.9%) saline and re-evaluate.
    - If SIADH is known or suspected, initial treatment should be fluid restriction to 1 L/day and use of 3% saline IV infusion (if symptomatic) or loop diuretic plus sodium chloride tablets.
    - Arginine vasopressin receptor antagonists (Vaptans) may be indicated for patients with euvolemic or hypervolemic hyponatremia, including SIADH, heart failure, or cirrhosis with ascites.
    - Correct hypokalemia and metabolic alkalosis secondary to vomiting with potassium chloride supplementation.

- o Overcorrection:
    - To evaluate for overcorrection, monitor serum sodium at 4-6 hour intervals until mild hyponatremia (about 125 mmol/L) is achieved.
    - To manage overcorrection, replace water losses and consider desmopressin (2-4 mcg IV every 8 hours) after correction by 6-8 mmol/L during the first 24 hours.

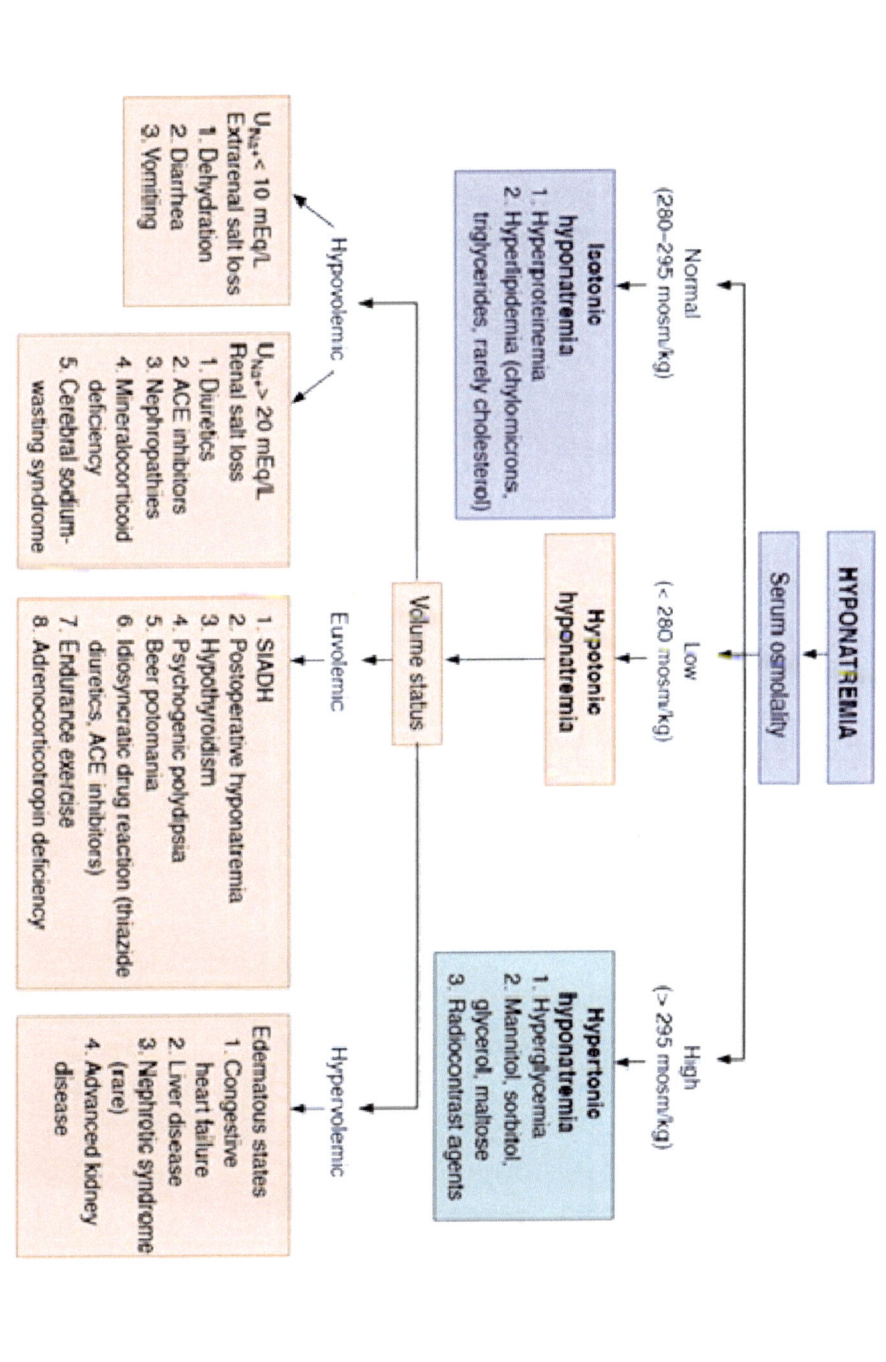

Metabolic Syndrome

- Metabolic syndrome is a cluster of commonly co-occurring metabolic risk factors associated with cardiovascular disease and type 2 DM, including:

    - Elevated blood pressure.
    - Atherogenic dyslipidemia.
    - Insulin resistance.
    - Central obesity.

- It is most common in overweight and obese patients, but it can occur in normal-weight patients.
- Risk factors include smoking, physical inactivity, and family history.
- The most common diagnostic criteria for metabolic syndrome is from the International Diabetes Federation (IDF) Task Force on Epidemiology and Prevention and the American Heart Association/National Heart, Lung, and Blood Institute (AHA/NHLB) and requires 3 of the following 5 criteria:

    - Triglycerides ≥ 150 mg/dL (1.7 mmol/L) or drug treatment for elevated triglycerides.
    - Fasting glucose ≥ 100 mg/dL or drug treatment for elevated glucose.
    - Reduced HDL cholesterol or drug treatment for reduced HDL:
        - In men, < 40 mg/dL (1 mmol/L).
        - In women, < 50 mg/dL (1.3 mmol/L).
    - Elevated blood pressure demonstrated by any of the following:
        - Systolic BP ≥ 130 mm Hg or
        - Diastolic BP ≥ 85 mm Hg

- - Antihypertensive drug treatment in a patient with a history of hypertension.
  - Increased waist circumference (as determined by population and country-specific thresholds).

- Management:
  - There is no specific treatment for patients with metabolic syndrome. The goal of treatment is to prevent cardiovascular disease and type 2 diabetes by managing the individual risk factors.
  - Lifestyle modification is the first-line treatment for all patients.
  - Advice a moderate-intensity physical activity for 30 minutes, preferably 45-60 minutes, ≥ 5 days/week.
  - In patients who smoke, smoking cessation is recommended.

- Complications include atherosclerotic cardiovascular disease (ASCVD), diabetes, and chronic kidney disease.

Hyperthermia Vs Hyperpyrexia

- Hyperpyrexia is an extreme elevation of body temperature which, depending upon the source, is classified as a core body temperature greater than or equal to 40°C.
- Hyperthermia is an example of high temperature that is not a fever.
- Fever, also known as pyrexia and febrile response, is defined as having a temperature above the normal range due to an increase in the body's temperature set-point (above 37.5 and 38.3°C).
- A "normal" core (internal) body temperature ranges from 35.6°C to 38.2°C in healthy persons.
- Hyperpyrexia differs from hyperthermia in that in hyperpyrexia, the body's temperature regulation mechanism sets the body temperature above the normal temperature, then generates heat to achieve this temperature; while in hyperthermia the body temperature rises above its set point due to an outside source.

Red Man Syndrome

- It is the immune system's adverse reaction to a given drug.
- The condition appears as red blotches or rash on the flushed skin from histamine release.
- It is commonly found on the back of the neck, it can also appear on the face and upper body.
- Vancomycin is the prime cause of this reaction.
- Other medications that can cause Red Man Syndrome include Teicoplanin, Rifampicin, Amphotericin B and Ciprofloxacin.
- Clinical manifestations include:

    o Redness or rash on back of neck, arms, upper torso or face.
    o Itchiness of the rash or red blotches.
    o Low BP.
    o Rapid heartbeat.
    o Nausea or vomiting.
    o Fever or chills.
    o Hives.
    o Muscle weakness.
    o Dizziness or fainting.

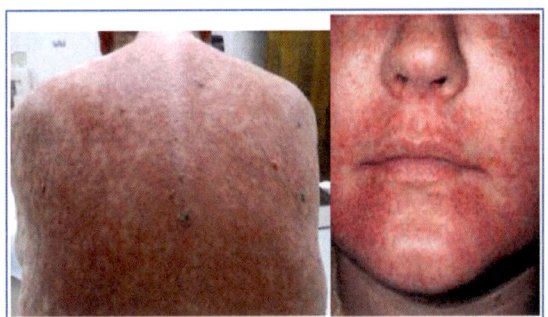

- There is no specific therapy for Red Man Syndrome, slowing the rate of the infusion is a good option.
- To be effective, Vancomycin is usually administered by IV injection, and it is imperative that this be done slowly, over a 60 minutes time period. If done too quickly, it can cause a mast cell degranulation, an inflammatory process in which certain cells release secretory granules

in response to a perceived invasion. This results in a reaction such as Red Man Syndrome. This can also happen if Vancomycin is taken orally.
- Antihistamines are often administered to treat any effects or symptoms of the reaction.
- To avoid a reaction to Vancomycin and the Red Man Syndrome effects, some patients are given Hydroxyzine before their infusion. This medicine has also been shown to help lessen the itchiness and the redness in patients that experienced the effects.
- Some patients can also be treated with 1 g of Diphenhydramine before their first dose of Vancomycin. This usually given over an hour-long time period.
- Red Man Syndrome is treated as a reaction or side effect rather than a diagnosis of a disorder.
- It is vital to observe a patient for the signs and symptoms of this particular syndrome after being administered specific antibody drugs, especially Vancomycin.

Insomnia

- Insomnia is the most common sleep disorder.
- Insomnia is defined as inadequate or poor-quality sleep characterized by one or more of the following: difficulty falling asleep, difficulty maintaining sleep, waking up too early in the morning, or sleep that is not refreshing.
- Acute insomnia is period of insomnia lasting between 1 night and few weeks.
- Chronic insomnia refers to sleep difficulty occurring at least 3 nights per week for 1 month or more.
- Insomnia may be associated with specific sleep disorders, including RLS, periodic limb movement disorder, sleep apnea, and circulation rhythm sleep disorders.
- Primary insomnia occurs in the absence of the previously mentioned conditions.
- The etiology of insomnia involves a combination of genetic, environmental, behavioral, and psychological factors which result in hyperarousal.
- Clinical manifestations include:

  o Daytime symptoms such as fatigue or low energy sleepiness or napping, and cognitive difficulty affecting attention, concentration, or memory.
  o Total sleep time < 6.5 hours.
  o Latency to sleep > 30 minutes.

- Management:

  o When the insomnia persists beyond 1 or 2 nights or becomes predictable, treatment should be considered.

- o Advise god sleep hygiene including regular moderate exercise and avoidance of caffeine and alcohol for several hours before bedtime.
- o Pharmacologic treatment is usually effective, especially short-acting hypnotics.
- o Chronic insomnia may be more difficult to treat. Because chronic insomnia is often multifactorial in etiology, a patient may need multiple treatment modalities, including medication (antidepressants, antihistamines, melatonin) and behavioral therapy.
- o Psychological and behavioral interventions (such as stimulus control therapy and relaxation training) are recommended for treatment of chronic primary and comorbid (secondary) insomnia.

- Complications include cognitive decline, reduced quality of life, hypertension, increased likelihood of receiving disability benefits, work absenteeism, and traffic accidents.

Sleep Apnea

- Obstructive sleep apnea (OSA) is a sleep disorder characterized by repetitive complete or partial (hypopnea) upper airway obstructions despite respiratory effort causing repetitive arousals and sleep fragmentation.
- Apnea is the complete cessation of airflow for > 10 seconds.
- Hypopnea is a partial airflow obstruction.
- The apnea-hypopnea index is the number of apneas and/or hypopneas per hour of sleep as measured by polysomnography as part of a sleep study.
- During an obstructive apnea event, alterations in intrathoracic pressure cause systemic and pulmonary arterial hypertension and sympathetic activation. This can lead to chronic and sustained systemic and pulmonary hypertension, arrhythmias, and associated complications.
- Risk factors for OSA include obesity, large neck circumference, snoring, male sex, and older age.
- Clinical features include:

    o OSA is most commonly associated with snoring, daytime sleepiness, and obesity but occasionally presents with insomnia.
    o Physical exam findings associated with OSA include:

    - Modified Mallampati score 3-4 (low visibility of posterior pharynx when patient opens mouth).
    - Retrognathia or increased overjet (top incisor teeth ahead of bottom incisors).
    - Lateral peritonsillar narrowing.
    - Macroglossia.
    - Tonsillar hypertrophy.
    - Elongated or enlarged uvula.
    - High-arched or narrow hard palate.

- Nasal abnormalities (polyps, deviation of septum, turbinate hypertrophy).

- Diagnosis:

  - In-lab polysomnography (PSG) is the recommended diagnostic test for OSA and for excluding other non-obstructive causes for sleep disturbance.
  - The diagnosis of OSA is confirmed if the number of obstructive events (apnea, hypopnea, or respiratory event-related arousal) on PSG is > 15 events/hour, or > 5 events/hour in the context of specific symptoms such as daytime sleepiness, gasping or chocking, or bed partner describing loud snoring or breathing interruptions during sleep.
  - OSA severity is defined as:
    - Mild for respiratory disturbance index (RDI) ≥ 5 events/hour and < 15 events/hour.
    - Moderate for RDI ≥ 15 events/hour and < 30 events/hour.
    - Severe for RDI ≥ 30 events/hour.
  - Continuous positive airway pressure (CPAP) titration can be performed during in-lab PSG or at home with autotitration. Autotitration is not recommended as a method for diagnosing OSA.

- Management:

  - Weight reduction is recommended in all overweight and obese patients with OSA.
  - CPAP is the treatment of choice for moderate-to-severe OSA as it has been shown to improve quality of life, reduce excessive daytime sleepiness, decrease motor vehicle accidents, and improve comorbid conditions such as heart failure or COPD.
  - Oral appliances including mandibular advancement devices and tongue retaining devices are indicated for use in patients with mild-to-moderate OSA who prefer oral appliances to CPAP, are

- unresponsive to CPAP, are not candidates for CPAP, or who fail behavioral measures such as weight loss and repositioning.
  - Medications such as modafinil may improve daytime sleepiness and may be used in conjunction with CPAP therapy or mandibular advancement devices in selected cases but not as sole therapy for OSA.
  - Surgical procedures, such as uvulopalatopharyngoplasty, may be used to reshape or open up the airway in patients with mild OSA with surgical correctable severe obstructing anatomy, but the degree of benefit for clinical outcomes is unclear.
  - A follow-up polysomnography should be performed to assess the effectiveness of CPAP after substantial weight loss (for example, 10% of body weight) or if there is insufficient clinical response.

Restless Leg Syndrome (RLS)

- RLS is a neurologic disorder characterized by unpleasant sensations in the legs or feet that are temporarily relieved by movement.
- Symptoms are worse in the evening, especially when a person is lying down and remaining still.
- The sensations cause difficulty falling asleep and are often accompanied by periodic limb movements.
- RLS may be either primary (idiopathic) or secondary to various conditions, such as iron deficiency, chronic renal insufficiency, pregnancy, or neuropathy.
- Diagnosis:

    o In adults and adolescents ≥ 13 years old, the diagnosis is made clinically by the presence of all of the following:

    - Urge to move legs often accompanied by an unpleasant feeling.
    - Onset or worsening of symptoms when at rest.
    - Partial or complete relief by movement for as long as movement continues.
    - Circadian pattern with high frequency of occurrence in evening and at night (often interferes with sleep).

    o Additional criteria in children aged 2-12 years include either of:

    - A description of leg discomfort by child in age-appropriate words.
    - At least 2 of the 3 of age-appropriate sleep disturbances, biologic parent or sibling with "definite" RLS, and periodic leg movements of sleep.

- o Consider testing of patients with RLS for iron deficiency, folate deficiency, vitamin B12 deficiency, diabetes, kidney disease, and thyroid dysfunction.

- Management:

  - o Exercise may have some benefits for patients with RLS, but data demonstrating efficacy is very limited.
  - o Patients with moderate-to-severe disease with negative impact on their lives either every day or on most days of the week should be treated daily.

    - Non-ergot-derived dopaminergic agonists, pramipexole starting dose 0.25 mg, maximal dose 0.75 mg or ropinirole starting dose 0.125 mg, maximal dose 4 mg orally once daily 2 hours before bedtime are considered first-line medication therapy.
    - Gabapentin starting dose 300 mg, maximal dose 2,700 mg or pregabalin starting dose 25 mg, maximal dose 300 mg may be considered for second-line therapy, or as primary treatment if there are associated pain symptoms.

Preoperative Risk Assessment

- The Revised Cardiac Risk Index (RCRI), also known as the Goldman Cardiac Risk Index, is a widely used tool to evaluate perioperative risk of fatal or nonfatal cardiovascular events following noncardiac surgeries.
- The components of the RCRI are:

    o History of ischemic heart disease.
    o History of heart failure.
    o History of stroke.
    o Insulin-dependent diabetes mellitus.
    o Preoperative serum creatinine > 2.0 mg/dL.

Indications of Magnesium Sulfate

- Hypomagnesemia.
- Toxemia of pregnancy (indicated to prevent seizures associated with pre-eclampsia, and for control of seizures with eclampsia).
- Torsades de Pointes (polymorphic ventricular tachycardia).
- Preterm labor (used as tocolytic to stop preterm labor).
- Acute nephritis in pediatrics.
- Exacerbations of acute asthma in the ED.
- Severe brain problems (encephalopathy).

Classifications of Antibiotics

- Some antibiotics are bactericidal, meaning that they work by killing bacteria. Other antibiotics are bacteriostatic, meaning that they work by stopping bacteria multiplying.
- The main classes of antibiotics are:
- *Beta-Lactams:*

    o Penicillins:

    - Penicillins are generally bactericidal, inhibiting the formation of the bacterial cell wall.
    - The main side effect is neurotoxicity.

    o Cephalosporins (bactericidal):

    - First-generation:

        ❖ E.g., Cefazolin, Cephalexin.

    - Second-generation:

        ❖ E.g., Cefuroxime, Ceforanide.

    - Third-generation:

        ❖ E.g., Ceftriaxone, Cefotaxime.

    - Fourth generation:
        E.g., Cefclidine, Cefepime, Cefquinome.
- *Macrolides:*

- They are mainly bacteriostatic agents.
- Examples include:
  - Azithromycin, Clarithromycin, Erythromycin.

- *Fluoroquinolones:*

  - They are bactericidal agents.
  - They should be avoided when possible in pregnant women and children.
  - Examples include:
    - Ciprofloxacin, Levofloxacin.

- *Tetracyclines:*

  - They are bacteriostatic agents and work by inhibiting the bacterial protein synthesis.
  - Examples include: (Doxycycline, Minocycline).

- *Aminoglycosides:*

  - They are bactericidal and bacteriostatic.
  - Examples include: (Gentamicin, Neomycin, Streptomycin).

Mentzer Index

- The Mentzer index, is said to be helpful in differentiating iron deficiency anemia from beta thalassemia.
- If a CBC indicates microcytic anemia, the Mentzer index is said to be a method of distinguishing between them.
- The index is calculated by dividing the MCV over RBC.
- If the MCV / RBC less than 13, thalassemia is said to be more likely.
- If the result is greater than 13, then iron deficiency anemia is said to be more likely.

Antidotes

Agent	Indication
Activated charcoal with sorbitol	Used for many oral toxins
Theophylline	Adenosine poisoning
Beta blocker	Theophylline
Atropine	Organophosphate and carbamate insecticides
Pralidoxime chloride (2-PAM)	Organophosphate insecticides, followed after atropine
Calcium chloride	Calcium channel blockers, Black widow spider bites
Calcium gluconate	Hydrofluoric acid
Chelators such as EDTA	Heavy metal poisoning
Cyanide antidote (hydroxocobalamin or vit B12)	Cyanide poisoning
Cyproheptadine (1st generation antihistamine)	Serotonin syndrome
Deferoxamine mesylate	Iron poisoning
Digoxin Immune Fab antibody	Digoxin poisoning
Diphenhydramine hydrochloride and benztropine	Extrapyramidal reactions associated with antipsychotic
Ethanol or fomepizole	Ethylene glycol poisoning and methanol poisoning
Flumazenil	Benzodiazepine poisoning
Glucagon	Beta blocker and CCB poisoning
100% oxygen or hyperbaric oxygen therapy (HBOT)	Carbon monoxide and cyanide poisoning
Idarucizumab	Reversal of Dabigatran etexilate
Leucovorin	Methotrexate and trimethoprim
Naloxone hydrochloride	Opioid overdose

N-acetylcysteine	Paracetamol (acetaminophen) poisoning
Octreotide	Oral hypoglycemic agents
Protamine sulfate	Heparin poisoning
Prussian blue	Thallium poisoning
Physostigmine sulfate	Anticholinergic poisoning
Pyridoxine	Isoniazid poisoning, ethylene glycol
Phytomenadione (vit K) and fresh frozen plasma	Warfarin poisoning and indanedione
Sodium bicarbonate	ASA, TCAs with a wide QRS
Succimer, Dimercaptosuccinic acid (DMSA)	Lead poisoning

Snjad-Sakati Syndrome (SSS)

- It is also known as Middle East Syndrome, is a rare autosomal recessive disease.
- It is caused by mutations or deletions in the TBCE gene of chromosome number 1.
- The condition is characterized by a triad of:

    o <u>Hypoparathyroidism</u>: with episodes of hypocalcemia, hypocalcemic tetany, and hypocalcemic seizures.
    o <u>Growth and mental retardation</u>: mainly as a consequence of repeated seizures.
    o <u>Dysmorphism</u>: including long narrow face, deep-set and small eyes, beaked nose, large and floppy ears, small head (microcephaly), thin lips with a long philtrum, small hands and feet.

- It is also characterized by low birth weight due to IUGR.
- Diagnosis is mainly clinical.
- Supportive treatment in the form of vitamin D and growth hormone supplementation is often offered to patients suffering from SSS.